FILLING THE GAPS

Discover What Prevents You From Achieving Extraordinary Results

The Proven Method for Injury Prevention, Recovery and Improved Performance

by **Michael Gee,** ATC

Praise for *Filling the Gaps*

"Wow, the program is amazing!! I was experiencing excruciating, persistent lower back pain for approximately 3 weeks, disabling me to walk pain free or stand upright. I thought the pain could be remedied by going to the gym, by performing light exercises and stretching. To my dismay, this alleviated little of the pain or the spasms. I reached out to Mike, who listened to my symptoms and put together a customized program. Once I completed the first series of the program very slowly, I immediately gained the ability to stand upright, and with a significant decrease in the intensity of pain. Mike is extremely knowledgeable and I have experienced first-hand, the results. His methods have demonstrated they truly work and what he has to offer is highly valued! Thanks Mike!" — **Satisfied Client**

"I had recently re-aggravated an old injury to my left ankle and required physical therapy. Throughout the following four weeks, I was in a boot and going to therapy three times a week. During this month of rehab, I was subconsciously compensating my weight to the opposite side. Once I was cleared to resume normal activity, I was working out and felt a sharp pain in my upper right glute and hip. For two months I walked around painfully, trying to avoid sitting down for longer than ten minutes. It was frustrating for me since I'm an athlete and live a very active lifestyle. One day when I was at my hometown gym, the ACM was introduced to me. I performed the assessment and my problem areas were pinpointed. I was prescribed a series of corrective exercises that I immediately started doing. The very first time I

did these exercises I felt relief. I could touch my toes and was almost completely pain free. I have since performed these exercises daily for almost two months and have been fully functional and pain free. If I ever have a day where I'm seated for an extended period of time I will do these exercises throughout the day to ensure my hip doesn't get bound up. I'm very thankful for the ACM and would encourage anyone who experiences pain to give it a shot. I'm very confident in the ACM's accuracy when assessing pain. If it worked for me it can work for you!" — **Seth Sharp, Athlete, Personal Trainer**

"I am so grateful for Mike. Most recently, I hurt my back (mid-back, right between my rib cage and hips) in a big way and could barely stand, sit or even breathe without being in complete agony. I was home alone with my three-year-old at the time, and it was just two days before Christmas, so there was no way I could spend the day lying down.

I called Mike, described my pain and injury, and he talked me through several exercises that helped me feel a lot better immediately. After doing the exercises for 20 minutes or so, I could stand and get through my day in a lot less pain. I continued to do the exercises several times a day for the next few days and was probably pain-free within four days.

Mike also helped me with another episode of excruciating back pain last year (lower back), the day before I was scheduled to fly cross-country for a family vacation. I called Mike and he created a set of exercises that enabled me to get through the flight and enjoy our vacation (though I had to do the exercises a few times every day).

It is really amazing what Mike can do over the phone, and I don't know what I would do without them. — **Ayn C.**

"*The ACM Fundamental Movement Assessment has changed my approach to training my athletes and clients. I've always tested some performance variables like VJ, SLJ, and agilities. I would also look at OHS pattern and push-ups, thinking I was assessing mobility and stability. While this assessment gave me a little insight into their general athleticism, it really didn't tell me much about stability or mobility. Sure, I would say, well, they can't OHS, heels come up, knees forward, elbows flex and arms come forward, or they can't do a full push-up and keep body straight, hips sagging, scapular winging, or their butt is in the air. What it didn't tell me was why.*

The ACM works in a manner that I can now begin to predict how they will score on each assessment from the way they moved in a previous one. There is crossover and integration in both the assessment and the corrective exercises so I can eliminate or confirm what my athletes are demonstrating through these fundamental movement patterns. The corrective exercises have such an immediate impact on these movements. It makes it easy for my athletes to "Buy In" and see what they "NEED" to improve so that they can optimize their training.

The ACM Fundamental Movement Assessment has increased revenue and improved customer satisfaction at ABSolute FiTness. Just by explaining the ACM to new members shows them that we genuinely care about their success, helping them understand that building a foundation of functional capacity will allow them to optimize their attempts at strength and conditioning, and their overall fitness. The first step in this Optimal Training Method is to start with the ACM Fundamental Movement Assessment. You will be able to upsell your new member and provide them with quality care and your expert knowledge. It is win-win, because even those that choose not to pursue the ACM now, typically will later. But, they will all feel your compassion and see the experience and knowledge that you can provide. **– Tim Zupancic, ATC, Owner of ABSolute FiTness**

Table of Contents

Dedication

*"What we know is a drop,
what we don't know is an ocean."*

– ISAAC NEWTON

To those who believe in the value of learning and have the courage to realize there is always more to discover.

It is my greatest ambition and intention that the knowledge and insights of this book reach those who need it the most and inspire those who have the ability to make the greatest difference in the lives of their patients and clients.

Foreword

BY LUCHO CRISALLE

I met Mike Gee 20 years ago. I remember being in Hawaii as support staff for a Tony Robbins event, and one of the breakout sessions was this "new method" to becoming pain free through postural alignment. Having degrees in Food Science, Human Nutrition and Exercise Kinesiology, anything related to movement and performance has always been a topic of interest to me. I was immediately intrigued by the method they were using to assess and correct people's postures and how quickly their recommendations had a positive effect not only on the subject's pain, but also on their performance.

After coming back to the mainland, I decided to go to the headquarters of the founder of this method, and that is where Mike and I became fast friends. At the time, I was a Registered Dietitian at Torrance Memorial Medical Center, where my rounds included the burn, intensive care, oncology and orthopedic units. After working in the hospital environment for five years, I decided to open my own private practice in Orange County, CA. As it turns out, our office was just a few blocks away from the company that Mike worked for as an injury prevention consultant. We got together for lunch and realized that we both had launched our own companies at around the same time and began to collaborate with each other.

Through the years, we have remained in contact, and I have seen Mike's system evolve by leaps and bounds. From the original postural alignment method that first brought us together, it has become a much more comprehensive system that assesses your body's function, mobility and alignment from the bottom up. The focus is on your joint function of either mobility or stability, as well as identifying which joints are compensating for the ones that are not doing their job as designed.

The beauty of this system is that it does not just stop at the "assessment," as other programs that I have seen in the health, wellness and fitness industries. Mike's program, ACM 360 PRO goes well beyond that. ACM stands for Assess, Correct, and Move. This is the only system that I, and many of my personal clients and family members, have used to correct our "dysfunction," to not only become pain free, but to also avoid future injury and improve performance at the same time. The key word here is CORRECT, which is what the rest of the other "assessment" programs are lacking. "Yes, I know I don't have XYZ range of motion…why and how do I correct it?" That has always been the question. ACM360 is the answer.

A specific example of the efficacy of his methodology is how Mike helped my wife, Lisza, after she threw out her back during an exercise class. She has been active all her life, teaching all sorts of sports and fitness classes ranging from swimming, skiing, Spin, aerobics, personal training and competing in martial arts, triathlons and figure competitions. Like many athletes, she thought that being in pain was just part of being an athlete. It was recently, during her mid 50s, that while training, a freak movement caused an extreme spasm in her lower back, rendering her virtually immobile. Having been married for 12 years, I have seen her have the same issue at least once every 12 to 18 months, and as stated above, we were both under the impression that it was just the way things go for athletes. Luckily, our relationship with Mike increased to a much higher level when we started collaborating in a master mind together a couple of years ago. This allowed us to become much more familiar with his methodology and system. Mike developed a program for Lisza to follow, and within one day she was no longer immobile and just a few days later she was able to complete a two-hour, straight-up hike to Camelback Mountain in Phoenix.

When it comes to performance, movement, stability and mobility, Mike has the unique ability to see things others can't and to instantly design a program based on the individual that addresses their specific dysfunctions and limitations, that shines a bright spotlight on the missing link to functional training. Through his certification program, Mike has established a clear step-by-step system to educate personal trainers, safety professionals, active release providers, chiropractors, physical therapists and athletic trainers to assess these dysfunctions, and through his software program, create corrective exercise routines that will allow them to help their clients at a level at which they have never been able to help them before. One of the great things about Mike is his passion for helping people feel better, do better and perform better, and because of this passion he does not exclude anyone. So even if you are not in the health, fitness and wellness industries, and are just interested in learning and implementing the Gee Method for your own benefit, his programs are the best place to immerse yourself in amazingly applicable knowledge that will impact your life in the most positive way, now and into the future.

I have been in the health and fitness industry and "world" for over 30 years, and as you can imagine, have come across many experts in the field, both knowledgeable and not so knowledgeable. Mike's knowledge, his ability to apply, teach and convey that knowledge, only pales in comparison to his passion on the subject, and his passion for helping others. We would often chat about the horrific (sometimes humorous) things we would see people do in the gym, and those conversations would always lead to, "Mike, you should write a book about this... and how to fix it." I am ecstatic that he finally did write a book on it and that he did not do so to impress anyone, but more notably, to impress upon them the importance of resilience, focus, education and never giving up.

In this book, Mike shares with you the struggles, pain and suffering that he endured as an active kid and as a young athlete, along with the doors that were shut in front of him that eventually led him to developing his method and sharing it with the world. You will read how it all starts with taking responsibility for your own well-being and having a "don't take no for an answer" mindset, followed by the empowerment fueled by education that eventually leads you to a paradigm shift where all is possible. He shares with you how pain and discomfort are truly signs more than symptoms. They are signs your body is giving you to let you know that there is a dysfunction, and by reading this book and implementing Mike's programs, you will now have the knowledge to identify that dysfunction and more importantly, the step-by-step instructions on how to correct it in record time without going under the knife.

My father was an orthopedic surgeon, so I have nothing against surgery; however, surgery should ALWAYS be the LAST RESORT. The Gee Method and the ACM system are your keys to a better life; a life without pain, a life with higher performance and in many cases, a life without surgeries. Some of the brilliant gems of wisdom he shares with you include, "If you are not functional, functional training will not fix you." It never ceases to amaze me, seeing trainers on the gym floor having their clients perform squats with plates under their heels because they have a lack of ankle mobility, when in reality they should be assessing their clients for functionality first and foremost. There is a difference between Functional and Fundamental Movement patterns, and Mike clearly explains this difference in a way no one else can.

I am so excited that this book is now available, as it will benefit professionals in the health and fitness industry, physical therapists, athletic trainers, massage therapists, chiropractors, ART providers, yoga and Pilates instructors and personal trainers. It is also for the layperson who just wants to be free from pain and improve their performance. In addition, it will help countless numbers of young and old who are now slaves to their electronic devices that cause their heads and shoulders to cave and lean forward making them look like human question marks, and those office desks, cubicles and other modern comforts that do nothing more than erode good posture, erasing the fundamental and functional abilities that we are all born with and deserve. Finally, there is a solution, and the solution is readily available for those who choose to take responsibility, take control of their mindset and become empowered by applying the knowledge they will find within the pages of this book and many of Mike's programs.

Who Should Read This Book and Why?

*"The good life is one Inspired by love
and guided by knowledge."*

—Bertrand Russell

One day, while working at one of the large corporations I consult with, an employee came to me very concerned about his 14-year-old daughter. He explained to me that she had been going to physical therapy over the past three months for pain in her left hip. She was not getting better, and the doctor said surgery was the only option, since physical therapy didn't help her improve. Desperate to help his daughter, he wanted to know if there was anything I could do. I told him, "I have no idea, but why don't you bring her in and we'll see what's going on?"

When I met Jordan, she was a very outgoing and energetic 14-year-old with a smile from ear to ear. It was apparent that the pain in her hip, the failed attempts in physical therapy and an impending surgery had her very confused and concerned. She explained all about what she was feeling and what she had been working on with the physical therapists.

Her rehabilitation was focused on hip strength, specifically lateral gluteal strength, Gluteus Medius to be exact. Upon initial observation it appeared that Jordan was very weak, because when she tried to squat, both of her knees rotated inward. This observation led to the assumption that her hips and glutes were weak and needed to be strengthened. The physical therapist hammered her with every "glute" exercise out there; side steps with bands, clam shells, outer thigh lifts, et cetera.

I knew one thing for certain. If her "problem" was glute or hip weakness, then 12 weeks of physical therapy, with a central focus on strengthening this area, would mean Jordan should have been fully recovered and jumping out of there. Since she was getting worse, I knew there must be something else that was missed in her assessment and treatment.

I took Jordan through the ACM Fundamental Movement Pattern Assessment and immediately discovered an extremely concerning dysfunctional pattern. Jordan had bi-lateral ankle mobility restrictions. She couldn't bend her ankle into dorsiflexion (pulling her toes toward her nose) past 0°. The normal range of motion of the ankle joint for dorsiflexion is 20°. In the ACM Assessment, we measure how far off the wall you can get your foot while touching the wall with your knee, keeping the heel down. The acceptable distance is 4 to 5 inches. Jordan's foot was less than a half inch off the wall. Any further away and her knee would rotate inward to compensate for the lack of ankle mobility.

Do you see where this is going? Read on...

I tested both ankles and sure enough, both ankles were completely restricted in dorsiflexion. For her to perform any type of squat or movement of the leg, she would avoid the restricted ankle mobility and just rotate her knees inward. This led to compensation throughout her entire kinetic chain, and her left hip was the area where it manifested.

To help her understand that the problem was in her ankle, not her hip, where everyone was focusing their attention, I had her attempt a squat with her feet flat on the floor. She performed three repetitions and during each attempt, her knees buckled in and she had extreme pain in her hip. Then I put her heels on a 2x4 piece of wood, raising her heels off the ground, eliminating the need for her ankle to move into dorsiflexion.

Jordan squatted down the first time a little reluctant, then stood up and tried it a few more times. She stopped after the third attempt and looked at me with confusion. I said, "What's wrong?"

She said, "My hip didn't hurt." A huge smile spread across her face.

What she didn't realize was that as she squatted down with her heels on the 2x4, her knees didn't buckle in. She squatted all the way down and had no pain during the movement. It was the perfect way for me to explain to her that it wasn't a hip problem, it was an ankle problem and nobody bothered

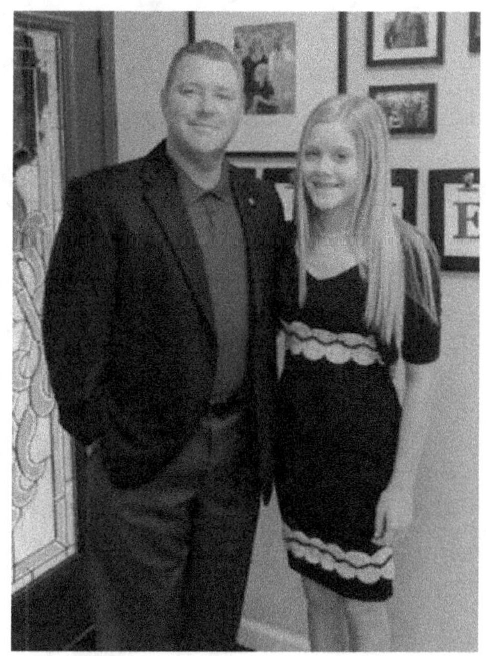

to look at her ankle mobility. It was why she hadn't been getting better all this time.

I am going to let you read what her Dad wrote me as a follow up to her progress for the rest of the story.

"Thank you so much for your support and taking time to see my daughter when I felt that her medical group had failed her. When I reached out to you, Jordan was 14. She was working hard on her school's water polo and swim team. Jordan began to suffer pain in her hip (no specific injury to relate it to that we knew of) and we immediately took her in to see a doctor. She was referred to physical therapy and after about 12 weeks was not getting any better. At our final appointment, a doctor commented that if she didn't get better she would probably need surgery. This scared Jordan and I couldn't believe that surgery was an appropriate answer when they didn't know the problem. When we came to see you, you diagnosed the source of her hip problem in about 5 minutes and recommended several exercises for her to begin doing. In about one week, the hip pain began to subside. After two weeks, the hip pain was gone and she felt 100% again. There's nothing worse than watching your daughter work hard through pain to stay competitive. She would get out of the pool many days in tears. Today, she is 16 and on the JV swim and water polo teams and very competitive. Thanks to you, she is strong, pain free, and wishes to pass her many thanks on to you."

So, is this book for you?

Tell me this – what if Jordan was your 14-year-old daughter? Wouldn't you want someone who could help her avoid a needless surgery and most likely a lifetime of disability and pain? Wouldn't you like to be the most effective practitioner you can be in order to help other Jordans?

There are countless people out there suffering in pain, having needless surgeries and who are confused and scared. As health care providers and fitness professionals, most of our patients and clients have underlying dysfunctions that could be limiting their progress and placing them at greater risk for pain and injury. It is our responsibility to ensure we have the knowledge, skills and expertise to really make a difference in their lives.

I encourage you all to join the ACM community, which can be found through my various social media sites at www.MikeGee360.com and visit www.ACM360PRO.com to get started with taking the next step in your education and professional development. I am certain the content in this book and the additional ACM Exercise Therapy Specialist Certification will offer tremendous value for your patients, your clients and your career.

Yes, this book is for you.

Let's get started.

One of the most important principles that I discuss in this book is
to not trust me, but to trust the method.

Introduction

"Mike, I can't help you. You need a knee replacement and you are too young for that. You'll have to wait until you are older and deal with the pain" the doctor said.

No one could ever have prepared me to hear those words at the young age of 26. I was in shock. Everything I had learned and believed had just been thrown out the window.

No more lifting? No more hockey? No more biking?

No more anything!

How was I going to be an effective therapist if I couldn't even fix myself? I questioned the industry in which I based my career. I questioned my education. Was there something I missed or was something else out there that I hadn't learned yet?

There were so many questions.

Although that doctor's statement eventually changed the trajectory of my life, the first question I had to answer was how I ended up there.

Growing up, we lived on top of a hill in a small town in Upstate New York. There was one tar and gravel road, no sidewalk and very little traffic. Because we lived in a very rural area, we had plenty of woods and a yard to play in, but to really go fast on our bikes, the street was the place to ride. We would go to the top of the hill and come down as fast as possible. A side effect of building our skills was falling, and we fell – a lot. I would say I became a master, and I had the constant scabs on my knees to prove it.

Aside from the crashes on the gravel road, we had a pond in our backyard which we used for a hockey rink. My buddy and I spent countless hours perfecting our slap shots and for me, perpetuating my knee problems. We used our knee caps as pads. I can still remember those searing sharp pains in my knee from falling on the ice.

When I was 10 years old, I saw my first doctor for knee pain. I remember the doctor telling me that I had bruised my cartilage and that there wasn't much I could do except take it easy. He gave me a note for my teacher, which allowed me to get up during class and perform an exercise to strengthen my knee. I got up and went to the back of the classroom to do the quad contraction exercise for three sets of 15 reps. I followed his advice. He was the doctor and must be right.

When I entered 7th grade, I started lifting weights. I was inspired by my cousin who was an up and coming bodybuilder in New Jersey and had won a Mr. Teen competition. I began lifting at the age of 12 and learned how to shape my body and build some serious muscle. For whatever reason, I was that one guy who loved doing legs. I was strong, and my legs were massive. I couldn't even fit into regular pants (later on, for my prom, I actually had to have my rental pants altered so they would fit).

At 15 years old, I did the long jump in gym class. When I landed, I felt a pop in my right knee. It hurt, and there was some swelling. I could actually feel a piece floating around and could move it side to side along my knee joint. I went to the doctor. This was before MRIs and special imaging techniques we have now, and he said I needed surgery. He said I had torn the cartilage in my knee and there was a loose body floating around.

Back then, especially in my little town, no one offered rehab or physical therapy. I had to learn some of these lessons the hard way. The day after surgery, still injected with pain killers, I thought it would be a good idea to get on my bike and ride around. Afterward, my knee swelled up to the size of a balloon. Ice? Who ever thought to put ice on an acute injury or post-surgery? I just hobbled around until the swelling eventually went away.

My sophomore year in high school, I was not allowed to play football because of the knee surgery, so I just sat on the sidelines watching my teammates. Keep in mind, I had surgery in the late spring the previous year, and the doctor wouldn't release me for almost a year from the time of surgery.

Within a few months, I was feeling okay. I still had pain, but I could bend my knee and got back into the gym as soon as possible. As I mentioned, legs were my favorite, and I started to really focus on lifting with a passion. I competed in my first bodybuilding contest at 16 years old and was one of the strongest guys in school. At the time, our mentors were the massively oversized bodybuilders we idolized on the covers of muscle and fitness magazines. Joe Weider was the only supplement company, and we consumed his protein powder like it was powdered sugar.

During those years, something began to happen. Aside from wanting to be freakishly huge like my idol, Tom Platz, who was known for his massive legs, I started to become intrigued with how the body worked. Those body building magazines were my first insight into human anatomy, and I really immersed myself in the articles that were related to the physiology and medical aspects of muscle growth.

At 18 years old, I was playing semi-professional football for a local team in our area that traveled throughout the northeast. I was lifting more than ever and enjoying the celebrity status that playing for the TC Jets gave us in our small town. We all knew it wasn't going to lead to anything more than bumps and bruises, but it was a fun time – except my knee had really started to bother me again.

At the end of the Jets' season, my knee didn't feel right. On occasion, it would lock up so I couldn't straighten it. I learned to slide my finger along the medial joint line to release it, but it was happening more and more often. I was fearful that it would lock up while I was playing, and it would get forced straight.

After seeing another doctor, it was decided that I needed another surgery.

My second surgery is really what helped guide me into my career, which I will explain later in this book. After surgery, the doctor sat me down and showed me the images from the arthroscopic surgery he had just performed. Not knowing what I was looking at, he explained it was the cartilage. Cartilage should be smooth, but the images illustrated huge fissures and "flaking" of the cartilage. Whatever he was showing me, it didn't look good. I remember him telling me in disbelief that he had never seen an 18-year-old's knee so destroyed. He said I had more arthritis than a 70-year-old man, and there were cracks in my knee cap. I specifically remember him saying, "Mike, if you don't stop playing all these sports and don't stop lifting, you are not going to be walking when you are 25 years old."

I returned home following surgery with so many questions, but at the time, no one could answer them. It was the late 80s. There was no internet and not a chance of seeing a physical therapist. I had to figure it out on my own. I was under the false impression that surgery had "fixed" my knee and things were fine now.

I got back into the gym and continued to lift against the doctor's recommendations. I was determined to out-mass my idol, Tom Platz. I was squatting over 425 lbs. and deadlifting over 500 lbs. If you are wondering about my bench – well, let's just say 325 lbs. was my max, and I could care less. I was a leg guy, and everyone knew it.

After a few years of "finding myself," I was accepted into college at The University of New York at Buffalo and was accepted into the exercise science program with a minor in sports medicine.

During those "finding myself" years there were a few constants in my life, the gym and the reminder of what that doctor told me after my second knee surgery. That reminder came in the form of pain. The more I lifted, the more it hurt. The stronger I made my legs, the more it hurt. It wasn't making sense to me at the time.

The education and experience I was gaining in the sports medicine curriculum was confirming what the doctor had told me. Arthritis was irreversible. Cartilage and meniscus did not regrow or repair naturally, and the degenerative process would continue.

By the time I was 26 years old, I was working at a physical therapy clinic in Denver, Colorado, which specialized in the spine and orthopedics. This was my opportunity to work alongside surgeons and some great physical therapists where I was convinced that I would learn how to help myself along with the patients I was treating.

Then one day, everything changed.

I was playing ice hockey at a local college club team. I traded my sports medicine expertise and guidance for the team in exchange for skating with them in practice and playing in non-league games. I still lifted and maintained my heavy squats and deadlifts, but I was living on Ibuprofen, taking 800 mg three times a day for my knee pain. At 26 years old, my knee was killing me.

I contacted one of the clinic surgeons for a consultation. I explained my history and what I was experiencing. I told him that I was doing everything I gave my patients to do. I told him how much I was squatting and lifting and that I still couldn't understand why I was "hurt." I assumed that the first two surgeries did the trick and tried to convince him that I needed another surgery to fix this problem. I was convinced that surgery was the only option since it helped so much in the beginning.

I will never forget his reaction and what he told me. He listened to my story, my concerns and eagerness to have surgery, then paused. He shrugged his shoulders and said, "Mike, I can't help you. You need a knee replacement and you are too young for that. You'll have to wait until you are older and deal with the pain."

I was speechless to say the least, and his news left me discouraged and depressed. Although there were still a lot of unanswered questions in my head, I knew I was facing the biggest decision of my life and knew that I had only two choices.

My first choice was to listen to the doctors. Up until now, they had all told me that I didn't have any other options. They said the degenerative process would lead to a sedentary lifestyle with a knee replacement in my future. It's nothing less than I had learned through my education and experience working in the Athletic Training and Physical Therapy fields. Who was I to question the status quo and challenge the medical model on which I had based my entire education and early career?

My second choice was the road less traveled. It would be the more challenging choice and would require me to dig deeper and learn more. I would need to immerse myself in the study of the human body, biomechanics and rehabilitation alternatives with really very little direction on where to start. The traditional medical model wasn't working for me; however, the education and experience I had gained made it very difficult to believe anything different. This choice also meant that I would be walking away from my current career path goals of working for a professional sports team as their athletic trainer.

The journey I chose has been enlightening, rewarding and challenging. Through the extensive time I lived in the gym, and my early career as an athletic trainer, I had many experiences. I reflected on these experiences years later, only to conclude that there were many gaps that needed to be filled, and the answers I found needed to be shared.

This book explores those gaps I found in the health care and fitness industries and establishes a philosophy and method for helping any patient or client achieve extraordinary results.

PART 1

The GEE Method

"The purpose of life is finding your passion, and giving it to others is what makes life meaningful."

–Mike Gee

"Mike, you've got to write the book, you've got to get this program out to the masses."

"What you have developed is incredible and everyone needs to know this."

These are the words that my clients and those closest to me have been telling me for years and something that I am extremely passionate about.

My days are filled with stories of people who are suffering with chronic pain, recovering from injury or surgery, or trying to improve their physical performance in sports or activities. What I have discovered seems so obvious to me, but I realize that from the stories I listen to and the advice many people get from others in the health care and fitness industry professions, there are big gaps that the method I've developed can fill.

It was 1:00 am on a Wednesday morning and I lay awake in bed. My heart was pounding and I couldn't fall back asleep. I woke up with a feeling of desperation and was experiencing a level of anxiety that I had never had before. I knew what was wrong. I've known it for years, but had been putting off. I knew that I wasn't going to fall back asleep and that I needed to take action immediately.

There was nothing more frustrating to me than to hear about injuries that could have been prevented, unnecessary or failed surgeries and rehabilitation practices that never advanced a patient toward independence. I was witnessing an industry trend in fitness that was misunderstood and guided by individuals who had limited knowledge and expertise who were having a significant negative influence on the general public.

My perfect storm had been building for years, and at 1:00am on that Wednesday morning in October, it hit me with the impact of a category 5 hurricane. I couldn't put this off any longer. The frustrations I had carried had escalated to a sense of urgency, and I knew many people needed what I had discovered.

I have dedicated my entire professional career to helping others achieve the same results I had with their physical performance and injury recovery goals. I developed a program that was successful and a method that transformed my life and the lives of my clients. I knew in my heart that my intentions were right and knew that I couldn't keep these secrets of success to myself any longer. There is nothing more rewarding to me than helping a person transform their own life from the grips of chronic pain and injury. I knew that when the sun came up that morning my life would change forever.

At 1:00 am that Wednesday morning, I began to write the mission and philosophy for what is now known as "The GEE Method." I still remember the sun coming up that morning, and after six hours of writing, the foundation to the GEE Method was complete. From that morning on, I have had one single mission – to deliver a method that will transform people's lives and offer an entirely different perspective for how the healthcare and fitness industries look at injury prevention, recovery and improving physical performance.

The GEE Method and the ACM System were developed out of necessity over the past 25 years, working with sports medicine, physical therapy, and fitness professionals. It was important to establish a philosophy and approach that would fill the gaps responsible for preventing someone from recovering from pain and injury and allowing them to achieve greater performance. This approach can be adopted by health care and fitness professionals who truly believe in the responsibility they have toward their patients' and clients' success.

The philosophy of the GEE Method is founded on three significant principles to achieving success in any area of life. These principles are essential to establish with every patient and client you are working with if you are going to be effective at helping them. It has taken me nearly a lifetime to understand how each of these principles played a role in the recovery of my knee pain and the many other injuries I sustained. Applying these principles in my life has been one of the biggest challenges and also the greatest reward.

Guiding Principle 1: You must take 100% responsibility.

Guiding Principle 2: You must commit and be willing to do whatever it takes to improve.

Guiding Principle 3: You must take massive action.

These principles appear simple, but they are not easy for some patients or clients to embrace. If you examine your own failures and successes, you will begin to recognize that each one of these three principles was responsible. The successes in your life were a direct result of taking responsibility for what you can achieve, you did whatever it took to make it happen and you took the necessary action toward that goal. Your failures can be viewed the same way and are the result of lacking one of these three principles in your pursuits.

As health care providers or fitness professionals, it is important to recognize which area your patients or clients may be struggling with and take the necessary actions to help improve their mindset towards their objectives.

Let's examine each one of the three principles for success as it relates to injury prevention, recovery and improving fitness and performance.

Guiding Principle 1

You must take 100% responsibility.

"With great responsibility comes great power."

— ADAPTED FROM SPIDER-MAN MOVIE

Now, I know most of you are thinking, "No, Mike, the quote is, 'with great power comes great responsibility,'" from the Spider-Man movie, when Uncle Ben says this to Peter Parker before passing away. I would say Uncle Ben was right, but if you just switch the statement around, as I have, you will begin to understand that taking responsibility for ourselves gives us great power. In taking 100% responsibility for the decisions and actions in our life, we actually become stronger and more capable. Without responsibility for ourselves, we allow circumstances and others to dictate what is possible, and that closes off any potential for growth and achievement.

It doesn't matter what has happened in the past. You must live in the present and focus only on what you can do now. There are many circumstances and events that are out of our control. The only thing you can control is how you react to the events, person or circumstances. I've found this to be one of the biggest challenges a patient or client will face in their efforts toward recovery from injury or improving health and performance. When we blame others or circumstances for our current conditions, we are allowing those people and events to determine our own outcomes. Although it may be easier to place the responsibility elsewhere, initially, we are slowly giving up our own power and creating dependency. In the long run, placing blame elsewhere will never help resolve your current situation or condition.

Blaming others is referred to as the "victim mentality." This may seem like a harsh statement, but listen, I understand pain, and I understand injuries. I have had six orthopedic surgeries, three broken bones and countless torn ligaments and muscles. I know what it feels like to be depressed and have no light at the end of the tunnel. I know what it feels like to live on Advil and Tylenol for the pain. For years, I blamed my conditions on genetics, other people and circumstances with no light at the end of the tunnel, but I wasn't getting the results I wanted and realized why. I wasn't being responsible for what I could be doing and instead it was easier to blame others.

We all go through different emotions when we are injured and in pain. It's just how long you stay in that place that makes the biggest difference in your recovery. During those dark times, it is easy to place blame on others or because something happened out of your control. The problem is that this mindset does not help empower you to begin getting better. The longer you refuse to take responsibility for where you are right now, the longer you will be in the same situation you find yourself in. For those who are overweight, out of shape and suffering the ill effects of poor physical conditioning and health, the victim mentality is most likely what is holding them back, too.

What I generally listen for when I work with clients is that regardless of how or what has happened, the person is focused on their recovery, not the causes of their injury or health conditions. A person who assumes 100% responsibility for their recovery or their health doesn't put that responsibility on their doctor, physical therapist or personal trainer. They don't blame others for taking too long or not working with them long enough. They focus on where they are today and put the past behind them. They may not know what they need to do or how it will happen, but they don't blame others for their outcome. It is our job to encourage them toward the possibility of change and healing, and the services we provide need to empower them into taking responsibility for themselves.

This may take time for some people because of what they have been told their entire lives about genetics or the X-rays and MRIs they've seen. They have learned to blame others or circumstances beyond their control, and as a result, they have begun to believe that change is not possible. We will discuss the two most important aspects to influencing change later in this section.

Just understand that as a health care provider and fitness professional, the approach you take with each patient and client will further influence the victim mentality or empower self-responsibility. *One of the greatest factors that determines your client's success, regardless of the services you provide, is whether they actually think it is possible to improve.*

Mike is a client of ACM and a college baseball pitcher whose fast ball breaks 90 miles per hour. According to his strength and conditioning coach, he is one of the hardest workers in the weight room, and he has pro potential.

The problem was that Mike was having lower back and hip pain along with multiple groin and hamstring pulls. His ability to perform at his highest level both on the field and in training was declining. Mike had been seen by his team trainers, physical therapists, chiropractors and pitching specialists to address his concerns. All of these professionals had various techniques and ideas for how to treat his conditions, yet nobody really focused on the root causes or provided sustainable results. Mike started to believe that nothing could be done to help him.

When Mike started working with ACM, we discussed many of his concerns and the most obvious road block he was having was his own belief that his injuries and his limited mobility was a genetic factor. He believed it was something permanent. Mike didn't understand or realize that his belief, what we refer to as a fixed mindset, was one of the factors holding him back. This fixed mindset or victim thought process is one of the first factors we focus on at ACM. If you do not believe you can get better, if you believe that something is permanent or if you do not own your own problems and take 100% responsibility for where you are now, we know you are less likely to improve from your concerns or conditions.

We addressed Mike's belief about genetics and helped him understand that genetics plays a factor in many physical conditions, however, his movement pattern dysfunctions and postural compensations were something he could change. Following the ACM Fundamental Assessment, it was clear to Mike that his genetic makeup was not the factor. We found asymmetries from one side of his body compared to the other. The dysfunctions that were identified were associated with his environment and training habits. Once Mike came to this realization, the road blocks to his improvement were removed. He has improved tremendously with a mindset of growth for his future.

Most people want to improve their current situation, yet lack the confidence and certainty that anything can be done. Years of pain, failed attempts with surgery, rehab, exercise or yo-yo diets make it very challenging to establish the 100% responsibility mindset for many patients and clients. Their lack of commitment is a result of being led down the wrong path, and as health care providers and fitness professionals this is where we can make the biggest difference in their lives.

Guiding Principle 2

You must commit and be willing to do whatever it takes to improve.

While determining where my clients are in their level of personal responsibility for their current health condition or injury recovery process, I also listen for how committed they are to getting better. I will ask them, "How important is this to you?" It would be safe to say just about everyone says, "It is very important." Who wants to be in pain or overweight, right? Being 100% responsible for your situation is very closely tied to how committed you are to doing whatever it takes to improve. You can't have one without the other.

Most people don't realize the effort it will take to achieve their expected goals and what level of commitment they must make. As health care providers and fitness professionals, we know the expected time frames for the recovery of certain injuries and fitness gains. We have created programs, services and products that misguide the general public into believing that their efforts and commitment can be minimized or delegated to others. "Just do these three exercises to fix your back pain," "Take this pill and lose weight," "8-minute abs," or "Lie down on the treatment table as I do the work."

A person's level of commitment must match their expected goals. There are no short cuts. It is our responsibility to direct our patients and clients to the actualizations of what is truly expected of them and the efforts necessary. When it's important enough to your patient or client, they will assume the right level of commitment, but they need to be educated toward what realistic goals can be achieved at their current level.

Determining a patient or client's level of commitment is sometimes straightforward. I work with many clients who suffer from low back pain, specifically herniated discs. It is sometimes a surprise to my clients when I discuss and question their lifestyle choices, specifically if they smoke or have diabetes. There is well-documented research that shows the negative effects on healing with smokers and diabetics.

Our body has an amazing ability to heal if you provide the right stimulus, nutrients, oxygen and blood flow. It is well-documented that smoking cigarettes reduces oxygen uptake and blood flow responsible for healing. If someone smokes and is serious about recovering from their injury, then the first thing they should do is quit smoking if they are ready to do whatever it takes. Gathering information about a client's current lifestyle choices helps me determine what level of commitment they are willing to make and how important their goals actually are to them.

Ironically, many clients are unaware of the links to their current condition or health status and their lifestyle choices, or they truly are not ready to make the commitment necessary for changing their current behaviors. Their expectation toward their goals must be in line with their commitment. If someone wants to recover from a herniated disc fully, they must make the commitment to do whatever it takes, including quit smoking. We will discuss behavior change later in this book.

For years, I was looking for the "quick fix" to relieve the knee pain I experienced. Surgery and Ibuprofen was what I believed were the answers. After being rejected for a third surgery and having gastro-intestinal irritation from the amount of Ibuprofen I was taking, I had lost hope. At that time, I believed I had been doing enough work for myself. I was doing the exercises I gave my patients to do, plus my legs were incredibly strong from all the weight lifting I was doing.

When I realized that I hadn't been taking 100% responsibility for my problems, I also knew I hadn't been doing enough to find the answers. I had been listening to everyone else tell me my condition was hopeless. I had to take my pursuit to the next level and immerse myself fully.

I haven't fixed my arthritic condition in my knees, but I have fixed my body mechanics, adjusted my diet and drink a lot of water to minimize further damage. I am able to live a very active lifestyle and at the time of writing this book I have completed three half marathons, and continue to push the limits of what my body is capable of with very little limitation and pain. I made a commitment to myself that if I had pain in my knee, it's nobody's fault but mine, and I was going to do as much as I possibly could to help myself remain active and pain free.

I truly enjoy helping people achieve results like I have; however that wasn't what I set out to do initially. In the beginning, I was committed to finding the answer to fix myself first! How is that for doing whatever it takes to achieve success? I became my own therapist!

When I discuss with clients why it's so important to improve their current situation, I dig deep, and have even had clients break down and cry. No, I'm not insensitive. I know that if my client doesn't understand their purpose or see that what I'm asking them to do is worth it, they won't commit to the work they need to do. *My job is not to get people better, my job is to help people get themselves better, and finding why it's important to them is the key to their sustained success.*

Motivation is short-lived, and most patients and clients will adhere to your program for a few days. Remember, they are used to a different behavior, and without constant motivation from you, they will slip back into the old behaviors that got them where they are. You can continue to be their cheerleader and give them daily pep talks to motivate them, but you must be careful with this strategy. One of the biggest mistakes health care providers and fitness professionals make in attempting to gain commitment from their clients is developing dependency.

Establishing the commitment for doing whatever it takes to achieve your goals must come from a personal deep desire. Goal-setting exercises and taking time with your patient and clients to establish their why and review on a periodic basis will ensure that you are creating that necessary sustainable drive your patients and clients need. Provide your clients with the knowledge and resources to help them understand their condition or situation and educate them toward what is expected of them to achieve the results they want.

Guiding Principle 3

Take Action

"Do or do not. There is no try."

— YODA

I suffered many big crashes in motocross racing and in one particular crash, I dislocated my shoulder. We had just started the race, and 12 guys were heading up a long hill at top speed, probably over 40 mph. The hill started to level off, and there were a lot of braking bumps going into the first turn. The racer in front of me lost control and crashed. I had no place to go but right into him, sending me flying through the air. My bike landed on me as I hit the ground. Immediately, I felt my shoulder "pop" and knew that I had dislocated it. I had to scramble to get to the side of the track before the other racers hit me.

I spent the next two months, every single day, trying to rehab my shoulder and still couldn't lift or move it. At that point, I knew my actions were not getting the results I expected, and I needed surgery. I came to find out that my entire rotator cuff and labrum were torn apart. Following surgery, I spent another two months rehabbing my shoulder, never missing a day, and there were many days that I did my rehab multiple times.

One day I came home from work and was pretty tired. I remember sitting on the couch, exhausted, and did not feel like doing my shoulder rehab program. I thought to myself, "I can miss one day, who's going to care?" That's when it hit me.

EXACTLY, who's going to care? Who cares if I achieve my goals of getting back on the motocross track? Who cares if I can do pull-ups again or have the same level of strength in my shoulder as I did before? Sure, people cared that I was doing okay, but they weren't calling me and knocking on my door making sure I was doing everything I could to get back. That was the moment I realized it's truly up to me to make this happen. I needed to continue taking action every day, so I got up and went into my exercise room and did my rehab.

My first race back, which was about five or six months following my dislocation, I beat every one of my buddies who had been racing the entire time. They couldn't believe it, but I took 100% responsibility for what happened. I didn't blame that guy for crashing or the track for being rough. I did whatever it took to rehab myself before and after the necessary surgery, and I took massive action EVERY SINGLE DAY. The day after my dislocation, I got on my spin bike and made a commitment that I would at least stay in as good a shape as I could during the time I was recovering. I road my stationary bike for one hour every single day! EVERY DAY. I was committed, and knew it was going to take massive action on my part to achieve my goal of racing again.

If you want to accomplish your goals and achieve anything in life, including recovery of injuries and getting healthy, you must take action. Sitting around thinking about it, making plans and dreaming is a good first step, but the only way to see results is by taking the necessary actions. *Your current situation and condition directly correlates to the level of action you have taken or not taken.*

One of the greatest problems that I have found in over 25 years of working in sports medicine and athletic training, is that most people wait until there is significant loss to their health before they take action. They ignore all the signs that are right in front of them until something happens, and then wonder how and why.

Being overweight is a risk factor for many health conditions. If you google "overweight risk of disease" you will see that there are 12 major health factors associated to being overweight. Do you really need to wait until a near-death experience or chronic disease to make a change and take action? The majority of people I've worked with over the years admit that they knew there were problems, but those problems hadn't gotten big enough to make it a priority. Unfortunately, when it comes to some conditions and diseases, waiting to take action may be too late.

The level of action necessary to achieve what you want must match your expectations. Not only must they meet the level of your goals, but they must be the right actions and produce results. Those results must be measurable and can have a tremendous influence on helping a client achieve the first two principles for success.

Julie is in her late 40s and has suffered with a congenital hip condition her entire life. She has hip dysplasia and has experienced increasing pain over the past years. This pain has limited her from exercising as she did when she was younger, and she is considering following the doctor's advice and having her hip(s) replaced.

When I first worked with Julie, she told me the entire story with repeated emphasis on the congenital condition and what the MRIs looked like. Julie was ambitious about getting out of pain and returning to an active lifestyle, but the pain limited her, or so she thought. What was limiting Julie was her belief that whatever she did would cause pain, because it did. The film reel would play with what she was told and knew about congenital hip dysplasia and the cycle of anxiety, worry and hopelessness prevented her from taking more action.

I knew in working with Julie that changing her mind about genetics was not the direction I could take immediately. She was pretty convinced about what the doctors told her and what she learned on her own. Getting Julie engaged and committed was not hard. She was in pain and frustrated that she couldn't even do simple stretching exercises on her own. I knew that I had to prove to her that regardless of the hand genetics played and what the doctors told her, there was something that could help.

I had Julie do two simple exercises, different from what she was attempting on her own. As she was performing the exercises, she was extremely reluctant to believe that there would be any difference in her ability to walk and sit. The next day Julie told me how excited she was that just those two exercises had such a significant influence on her pain with walking.

Julie was trying to take action, but not the right kind of action, which reinforced her belief that there was nothing that could be done, and surgery was imminent. Taking the right kind of action toward your goals is critical. You must have a way of measuring results and determining if the actions you are taking are producing the results you want. If not, you must change the path of action you are on with the same level of commitment.

As a health care provider or fitness professional, we must encourage our patients and clients to take action for themselves. Coming to you for a massage or what I call with some rehab programs, the "warm fuzzies" (electric stim with a heat pack), is not the kind of action that results in sustainable and extraordinary results. The programs and services we offer as health care providers and fitness professionals must empower our patients and clients toward taking the necessary actions for themselves.

"The Universe rewards those who take action."

– Dr. Phil

It is important to hold yourself, your clients and your patients to a higher standard. That standard is something that cannot be compromised. It is built on a solid philosophy that supports self-reliance and independence. That philosophy should ensure that the services and programs you provide your patients and clients will empower and engage them toward taking personal responsibility for their own health and fitness pursuits.

The integrity of the health care and fitness professions has been established on the influence we have and perceptions we are delivering to the general public. We have the opportunity and responsibility to direct those views and expectations in a direction that can transform patient care and influence a more proactive approach toward health and fitness.

We are either part of the problem or the ones who influence change. The GEE Method and the ACM System were developed to be a direction of change and influence for the health care and fitness professions.

All Practices Can Benefit

I have been on both sides of the treatment table throughout my life and have an empathetic understanding of what it feels like, both physically and mentally, to be injured, in pain and scared. I know what it feels like to believe you are broken and there is no light at the end of the tunnel. I've been treated by physical therapists, chiropractors, massage therapists and have had my fill of medical diagnoses and orthopedic surgeries. I've listened to the doctors, therapists and professionals offering their advice and learned to differentiate the guidance offered.

I've spent my entire life competing as an athlete and involved in various fitness endeavors to understand the demands for improving human performance. I've worked closely with personal trainers, yoga instructors and strength and conditioning coaches deciphering their methods and approach for achieving the highest potential. It's these personal experiences as an athlete and patient, and the insights I developed as a therapist that fueled my passion for developing The GEE Method and ACM System.

All disciplines of the health care and fitness industries have their own unique contributions, philosophies and approach to treating patients and working with clients. The physical improvements we all work toward achieving with our patients and clients came from the same anatomy, physiology and biomechanics books, lectures and teachings. We apply that knowledge and our specific skills in the direction of our focused profession with the ambition to achieve the same results, at least in theory, leaving our patients and clients a little better off afterwards, both physically and mentally.

Some work on one end of the health spectrum in treating disease, pain and injury, while others work on the side of the health spectrum of improved performance. The design and function of the human body is the only constant. Our knowledge and expertise is based on the foundation of human anatomy, physiology and biomechanics as examples. The understanding that, regardless of our patient or client's conditions, the focus is to return to, or improve from, their current state to that with which the parameters of the human design dictate. Simply stated, we know what the body is supposed to look like and how it is supposed to function and each of our disciplines focuses on improving what may be wrong.

One of the greatest gaps I've discovered in working with, and being treated by, the many disciplines in health care and fitness, was the lack of consistency and congruencies toward injury prevention, recovery and improving performance. The varying opinions, methods and approaches for the direction of patient care and performance enhancement can confuse anyone. The latest gizmos, gadgets, pills, procedures and techniques all promise to be the answer.

Many professions have lost sight of treating the patient or client versus treating the symptoms and pain influencing the wrong expectations and developing perceptions that inhibit and reduce the advancements of our professional industries. The career paths we have chosen in the health care and fitness professions bring incredible pleasure and reward, and they also come with a tremendous responsibility. We are held to a higher standard and need to be accountable for the programs and services we offer. As authority figures and subject matter experts, there has never been a more important time to establish a new paradigm for health care and fitness that influences positive behaviors both in our professions and in society.

The purpose of The GEE Method and ACM System is to connect each of the health care and fitness professions with a singular philosophy and approach that is consistent and complements each other. Founded on the principle of the human design and the direction for changing the perspectives in health care and fitness for both patients, clients and professionals, The GEE Method and ACM System will complement, or in some cases replace your current approach toward patient care or improving performance standards. Each of the health care and fitness disciplines will benefit from adopting an approach that focuses on the fundamental design of the human body.

Don't trust me. Trust what the ACM System is telling you.

I've spent years testing and perfecting The GEE Method philosophy and ACM System to be certain of its sustainability and effectiveness. I have applied the principles to my own life, as the foundation to my training and for the many injuries I've sustained and from which I've recovered. I've used the ACM System as the primary focus in working with the thousands of clients over the years to help them prevent and recover from injury and support their efforts in the most effective approach toward improved performance. I can say with certainty that The GEE Method and ACM System will give you an entirely new perspective for what you are currently doing and guarantee that your patients and clients are getting the most effective approach toward achieving their goals.

As I tell all my clients, "Don't trust me. Trust what the ACM System is telling you." To a larger degree, as health care providers and fitness professionals, reflect on your current approach and what your beliefs are about helping patients and clients achieve results. As you read through each of the points in the "Gap" section, allow yourself to be open to a new perspective, and get excited for the opportunities and possibilities that a new direction on your path may lead you. You will begin to trust what your own instincts are telling you about each of the gaps I've identified, and you may even discover more from your own experiences that you were unaware of before. My greatest ambition with this book is to open your eyes toward something that could change your life, and I guarantee will change the lives of your patients and clients for the better.

**The truth is right in front of us,
we just need to be willing to see it for what it is.**

"Trust is earned when actions meet words."

-CHRIS BUTLER

My life's purpose is to have an impact in this world that influences others to achieve the results I have achieved. Beyond injury recovery and sports performance, my mission is to empower health care and fitness professionals to embrace the necessary changes that truly impact our society, and to develop a community of like-minded professionals who share the values and goals of making a lasting change. If you are serious about providing the programs and services that empower others to achieve extraordinary results, and you are one who is ready to become a leader in an industry that is in desperate need, this book was written for you. It is my greatest pleasure to share how I view the world, both from my experiences as a patient, and as a therapist, and am confident that you will begin to embrace what is right, not what is easy and popular.

Together, we will be that light at the end of the tunnel for many to move toward.

A Changed Perspective

One of the most impactful courses I had to take in college was a class called critical thinking. We reviewed published research papers, looked for discrepancies and challenged the researcher's hypothesis, methods and procedures. This class helped me look at everything I was learning with a slightly different lens and ultimately led me to excel in the field of corrective exercise because of the new perspective I had gained through my years of personal and professional experiences.

Do you remember the Matrix movie, where Neo was offered the blue pill or the red pill? The blue pill would allow him to continue living in the current world he was familiar and comfortable with, the red pill promised to show him the truth about what the matrix was and would offer him a different perspective about his life. Stay in your comfort zone behind an illusion or discover that the world was very different, and although it may be challenging to face, you would know the truth.

Imagine you were a young college graduate looking for work in a very unique and competitive industry that only rewarded the best, and opportunities to work at the top level rarely came along. Imagine you had interviewed with a professional sports team and were immediately offered the position, only to learn that you needed to wait the weekend because they reluctantly offered the job to another young college graduate. Well, you might guess how the rest of the story goes – sitting around on pins and needles all weekend hoping this other candidate said no. The call came on Monday morning and sure enough, the other person accepted the dream position.

Fast forward one year and imagine receiving a call from this same professional sports team to learn that they had kept your contact information and were eager to offer you this dream position. You would be working at their rehabilitation facility and in charge of rehab for professional athletes. Well, you might guess how the rest of the story goes. Imagine this – I said, "Sorry, I need to decline the offer." This dream job with a professional sports team would have been a launching point to my career, and the salary would have been double or triple what I was currently making. Who in their right mind would decline such an opportunity and why?

Do you want the blue pill or the red pill?

If you choose the blue pill, you can continue believing that I lost my mind for turning down the biggest opportunity of anyone's career and go back to the illusion of the fame and fortune I lost. If you choose the red pill you will learn the truth as to how I could turn down such an opportunity and why this path, although challenging at times, was the right one for me.

One of the greatest challenges I've faced throughout my career as a health care provider was when I developed the intuition for seeing things from a different perspective. Through my personal struggles with my knee injuries, and the clients I worked with for years, I started to understand what it really meant to get better and that I was the one who had the responsibility to provide that for my patients.

This new perspective was like seeing the matrix for the first time. Everything looked different – I could now see through the illusions and knew I could not ignore my instincts and needed to follow my own path toward what I believed was the right way. Opportunities to move in different directions were plentiful; however, all of my decisions were based on the understanding of what I had grown to believe and the philosophy that I had developed.

These new perspectives I discovered came from identifying gaps in my education, experiences and the guidance and advice I had been given from an early age. These gaps that I continue to mention are also what hold your patients and clients back from achieving the results they expect, and you as a health care provider or fitness professional, are ultimately responsible.

The Gaps

The first gap that we will discuss – and one of the most important to understand and develop – is the belief structures of your patients and clients.

The Belief Structure Gap

"Circle the area that best describes where you have pain or are hurting." If you have been to a doctor, physical therapist, chiropractor, massage therapist or any professional treating pain, the initial assessment begins with you filling out a diagram of the human body similar to the one on the right, asking you to illustrate where your pain is located. I have seen many of these subjective pain charts filled in like it was a coloring assignment. Then we ask you to describe your level of pain on a pain scale. The focus in health

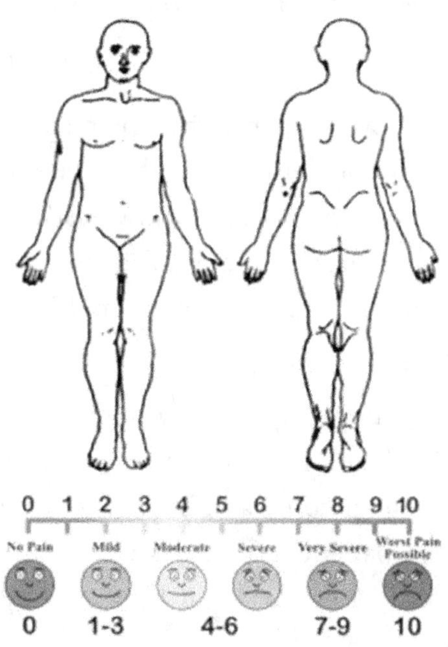

care with these charts is to gain a greater understanding of where people perceive their pain to be both in location and severity.

Usually during the initial assessment, we ask our patients and clients about their subjective awareness of their pain. This is where we give our patients and clients the opportunity to tell us their story. We write down these subjective findings in terms of how they were injured, how long it's been, what they are doing currently for treatment, when it hurts and find out if there is anything that relieves their pain.

One of the greatest lessons I learned through my professional career was to listen intently to understand my patients' and clients' viewpoint. Too often we listen to answer, not to understand. Early in my career, I found myself eager to speak and explain what I knew and what I could do to help my patients before really understanding what my patient was experiencing. It was only when I learned to listen to what my patients were telling me that I began to understand their perspectives, concerns and what may be holding them back.

What are your patients and clients telling you?

Everyone has their own specific story of what happened to them, how they got where they are and why they are looking to improve their current condition. Whether it's someone who suffered an injury, is dealing with chronic pain or wants to get into better shape, their stories are important for multiple reasons.

As I mentioned, in my early career I was listening to my patients explain where it hurt or what problems they were having. I would immediately begin going through my extensive mental database of human anatomy and injury recovery procedures. I would be quantifying the patient's level of tissue damage, recovery process and what I needed to do now for them. They told me where it hurt and why, what caused pain, how long it had been, what they had done up to this point – but they also told me so much more that I never paid attention to.

I recently was interviewed for a live Facebook promotion. During the interview, attendees wrote in comments and questions. Here is one of the questions that was asked:

> "Hip replacement? My left hip seems like I have bone on bone that seems to be what happens to people as they age. Very hard to walk because of that and both knees are going too. I'm well past 70. I BELIEVE!!!"

This gentleman was asking if the ACM program would be beneficial for those facing hip replacement surgery. The young clinician in me immediately would have thought of the degeneration of his hips, what stage had it progressed to, what did the X-rays and MRIs show, and also recognized that there was degeneration to his knees. Most health care providers would focus on these aspects of his concerns and have their own approach for addressing his degenerative hips and knees. In the past, I, too, would focus on the conditions and in the back of my mind know there was not much you can do for degenerative changes.

But what was he really telling me in his brief question? The first thing I now listen for with all of my clients is their belief structure. You see, to influence behavior change in anyone's life, there are two very specific characteristics or mindsets that must be present. *First, we must believe that we are capable or our approach needs to be geared toward helping our clients and patients believe they are capable of achieving the results they want. The second aspect of influencing behavior change is that you must believe that what you are doing is worth it.*

Looking back at the founding principles of the GEE Method, you can now begin to understand why taking personal responsibility is the critical first step in achieving the desired behavior change. To believe you are capable of accomplishing any goal, you first must believe you can, and to do that, you must take responsibility for what you can control.

Sir Richard Bannister broke the four-minute mile in 1954, a feat that most believed defied human capability. Many believed that running that fast would cause significant damage to the runner's health. Bannister's record would fall only 46 days later when John Landry would be the second man to break the four-minute mile barrier. Bannister would say that it wasn't the physical barrier, but the mental barrier that he needed to break. Today, a four-minute mile is expected and the standard for elite runners. Sir Richard Bannister went on to become an acclaimed neurologist, and his story of breaking the four-minute mile has become a lesson for many to understand how powerful mindsets and belief structures are in achieving the impossible.

As health care providers and fitness professionals, our primary responsibility should be to establish a growth mindset and influence positive behavior change with our patients or clients before we start working on them. The majority of conditions and problems people have are usually a direct result of the behaviors and actions they are currently taking. Our education, knowledge and training focus on how the body works, repairs and improves, and we use that knowledge to our best ability. Unfortunately, before your client or patient even comes through your door, they already have their beliefs toward what is possible and their motivations for doing so. If you do not focus on the belief structures that hold anyone back from achieving results, all the knowledge, training and education in the world won't have much of an impact.

This gentleman mentioned that "Bone on bone seems to be what happens to people as they age." That one comment told me more than his description of his concerns about his hips and knees. What is his belief structure? This man believes that it's an age-related process. There is nothing you can do about that and although his "WHY" is strong, the second characteristic in influencing behavior change – who wants to be in pain and not able to walk, right? His belief that this happens to older people tells me he doesn't believe he is capable, yet.

My initial conversation with this gentleman had nothing to do with his hip and knee concerns. Although I know his perspective and acknowledging that I heard his story is important, I also have learned that until your patient or client believes they are capable and they believe it's worth it, there is nothing you can do to help them. Our conversation centered on the "old age" perception he had. Many times I hear people telling me about their degenerative knee or hip and always relate it to "old age." The one question that stops them in their tracks is, "Isn't the other hip/knee the same age? Why aren't both sides having the same problems?"

It is critical to begin really listening to your patients and clients beyond their story. We must decipher their belief structure to identify what may hold them back from truly improving. When it comes to injuries, pain, health and fitness, what your patient or client believes is the reason for their current condition is truly what will hold them back or help them achieve the results they desire.

One of the greatest insights that I discovered holding me back in my knee recovery journey was the limited mindset that I had developed from an early age and was reinforced with my advanced education. I listened to my doctors, who I was expected to respect and hold to the highest standard. I didn't question their authority, and through my education I was learning the same thing they were telling me. I had too many reasons to not believe that getting better was going to be possible. It would take years for me to erase much of what I had learned and believed through small improvements and changes I was making.

The mindset and beliefs my clients have toward their own recovery process became my central focus. I knew from my own personal experience and from the thousands of clients I've worked with over the years that they need to believe they can get better and the process to do so will empower, engage and create independence for them.

Our own perceptions as to what is wrong with us and what we are capable of accomplishing are developed over a lifetime of experiences. From the time we are old enough to remember, our beliefs toward pain, injury recovery, health and fitness have been influenced by those who cared for us, what we watch on television, the internet and what we read in newspapers and magazines. Many of these influences have had negative effects toward promoting personal responsibility and self-awareness.

The traditional attitude toward health care and fitness is centered on the "what can you do for me" thinking. Patients and clients place tremendous responsibility and trust on what others can do for them and have been taught to believe this is the only way. The health care and fitness industry promotes an enabling perspective for others to believe that it is our responsibility to make you better. If something hurts, we expect our doctor, chiropractor or physical therapist to fix it. If you want to lose weight or get into shape, it is the responsibility of the personal trainer and strength coach to perform that task. If you are not seeing the results you expect, you blame the trainer or their methods and find another who is "better."

As heath care providers and fitness professionals we are ultimately responsible for enabling a fixed mindset or encouraging the growth mindset in our patients and clients. How we respond to and educate our patients and clients toward their health and fitness pursuits is the most critical interaction we have. The knowledge and skills we use in our practice and the services we provide must empower our patients and clients toward a growth mindset.

Cathryn Jakobson Ramin, the author of **Crooked: Outwitting the Back Pain Industry and Getting on the Road to Recovery,** discusses many of the problems she encountered while dealing with her own back pain. She spent nearly seven years researching the back pain industry, uncovering many of the misconceptions and misguided truths related to patient care and how the "system" works. She discovered many reasons why a back pain patient is like a revolving door to the medical community and the failed attempts at treating these patients.

In Cathryn's book, she discusses the advancement of imaging techniques like X-rays, MRIs and CT scans and how the results of these diagnostic tools leave patients with very little hope of believing they can recover. Having been diagnosed with a "condition" that is confirmed with these imaging techniques makes it very challenging for a patient to see any possibility of recovery.

These imaging techniques are valuable in many circumstances, but what Cathryn points out, and what most of the medical research suggests, is that the majority of us have abnormalities in the spine. It is very common to see compressed and herniated discs, arthritic changes and "crooked" spines in the majority of our society. Most of us have these abnormalities and are asymptomatic and can function through our daily activities. Then suddenly we "twist wrong" or "sleep the wrong way" and now we have pain.

It's believed that imaging techniques will reveal the source of the problem and much of the treatment is focused on that diagnosis. What is never discussed with these patients is that they have had arthritis and herniated discs long before they became symptomatic. Once someone believes they have a condition that is irreversible, it is very challenging to change that belief for them. It's very difficult to refute what these imaging techniques show us, however for those suffering with chronic pain and even acute injuries, it is important to always remember that there is a cause of this condition and that is what needs to be treated, not just the symptom. We will discuss more of this in the following section.

This is why, as health care providers and even fitness professionals, we need to be very careful with how we present findings to our patients, and although we should be honest with them, we need to also remember that we may be the cause of their limited mindset, belief structure and inability to get better.

To be effective at influencing behavior change, you first must be able to identify which mindset your clients and patients are coming to you with. The mindset for achieving results must be on believing it is possible, and without establishing this mindset, you will have a very challenging time engaging your patients and clients.

This section discusses how to identify limiting beliefs and fixed mindsets that you can begin to recognize with your patients and clients.

Mindsets

The ways we view our experiences and situations in our lives are dependent on two MINDSETS:

- The Fixed Mindset
- The Growth Mindset

The Fixed Mindset

A fixed mindset is one in which we view our life or situations in our life as set in stone, nothing will change. Our characteristics, our personality attributes, our losses, our failures, even our successes are nothing we have control of. It's a mindset of placing responsibility on something or someone else.

Examples of a fixed mindset:

- I have pain because of genetics. My parents have the same problem.

- My doctor said there was nothing they could do.

- The surgery I had was not successful. They messed me up further.

- I am too short or I am too tall (for whatever is being asked of them.)

- There isn't enough time in the day to do my exercises.

- Someone hit me while I was at a red light and messed up my back.

- I've gotten used to always being in pain. It's just how life is.

- Everyone who does "this" (insert what "this" is) has pain.

The Growth Mindset

A growth mindset is one in which we internalize the experience and try to gain insights toward how we can improve. We take 100% responsibility for our actions, and in return, we have to be willing to accept 100% responsibility for their outcomes, good or bad. This mindset provides that constant growth and a sense of certainty that you, and only you, are in control of your future where it is possible to improve.

- I have pain because I haven't been doing what I need to do for my health.

- There are many other programs that might help even though my doctor said they can't.

- I know I need to do more of my rehab following my surgery for it to help.

- I can't change how tall or short I am, but I can find a way around it.

- I have to manage my time better in the day so I can get to my exercises.

- I was in a car accident and know that I need to pay closer attention to how others are driving.

- I've been in pain for a long time, but it must have something to do with what I'm doing wrong.

- I am getting pain doing (XYZ) because I don't know how to do it more effectively.

As you interact with others, it will start to become even clearer whether a person is coming from a fixed mindset or a growth mindset. A simple question like, "How are you doing?" can reveal one's own mindset.

- **Fixed Mindset:** "I'd be better if the weather wasn't so bad."

- **Growth Mindset:** "Looking forward to getting caught up on things during this bad weather."

The fixed mindset response to your questions implies that it's the weather that is causing this person to not be having a great day. They see the environment and the things that happen to them as the reason they are unhappy or unfulfilled. The growth mindset response sees possibility and opportunity in every situation.

Let's look at another example to the same question, "How are you doing today?"

- **Fixed Mindset:** "I'd be better if I could lose 20 lbs."

- **Growth Mindset:** "Excited to get started and lose 20 lbs."

One statement implies that their life would only be better "if" they could lose 20 lbs. The extra 20 lbs. they are carrying around may be having an impact on their life, but it's the use of the word "if." It imposes even more challenges. A follow-up question should be, "Why can't you lose 20 lbs.?" A person with a fixed mindset will have another reason they can't lose the weight. On the other hand, the growth mindset person sees the 20 lbs. of weight loss as an exciting adventure. They know it's possible and are more willing to do what it takes to accomplish it.

Consider your own mindset centered on the rehabilitation or fitness programs you provide your patients and clients. I have worked in the health care and fitness industry for over two decades and met amazing therapists and trainers with some of the most positive and growth mindsets. I have also met many who share a fixed mindset and limit their own abilities to help their patients and clients succeed.

- **Fixed Mindset:** People just don't care about their health or fitness.

- **Growth Mindset:** I need to work harder on motivating people to care about their health and fitness.

- **Fixed Mindset:** No matter what exercise program I give my patient/client, they just don't like it.

- **Growth Mindset:** I need to listen more carefully to what my client's goals and motivations are to really understand how I can help them.

- **Fixed Mindset:** I've tried to introduce corrective exercise programs to my clients and they just don't want them.

- **Growth Mindset:** My clients don't understand the importance of corrective exercise, and I need to do a better job explaining the benefits to them.

Understanding mindset patterns is similar to what you already know from the old cliché, a glass half full or a glass half empty. It holds true that people who see the glass as half empty tend to be working in the Fixed Mindset pattern while those who see the glass as half full are using a Growth Mindset pattern. Paying close attention to what someone is saying, regardless of the situation or their story, you will start to hear the mindset through which they view their world.

Awareness of a person's mindset patterns will be one of the greatest insights you can have toward understanding their belief systems and how they think of themselves. Knowing how a person sees the world, and where they view themselves in that world, will help you understand if you need to spend more time helping shift their mindset toward possibility before you can truly help them achieve the results they want.

Your programs and services must empower your patients and clients and give them a foundation that they believe is possible and worth it for them.

Filling the Belief Structure Gap

They come through our doors for a reason.

Many years ago, working for a private clinic, I had a discussion with my boss about a particular client. This client, for all intents and purposes, was the client from hell, at least that is what all the therapists thought of her. She was challenging to work with because she felt that she was different, special and what applied to others didn't apply to her. Her focus was all over the place and she was not compliant with her exercise program on her own. None of the therapists wanted to work with her, and she would single me out as the only one she wanted to work with.

We didn't have our own client list. Who we worked with was dependent on the schedule of the day and clients were paired randomly with therapists. We did this for a very specific reason – to avoid client dependency on just one therapist.

My boss explained to me after listening to many therapists complain about this particular client that, "Every client who comes through that door comes with different problems and for different reasons." It was our responsibility to determine what that client needed and offer our help. He never really explained how, but I started to learn that some clients needed to shift their mindset toward growth, some needed to believe in the potential for their bodies to heal, and some were just ready to get started.

I believe the reason this client wanted to work with me was because I listened to her. I didn't dismiss her sarcasm or lack of focus as disrespectful and closed off. She came to us for help, and although the progress with her program was slow due to her disbelief about what she was capable of, she still came and was committed. I recognized that the majority of the time I worked with her needed to be focused on listening to her concerns and limiting beliefs and to offer new directions and paths that would help her change the current perspectives she had.

The GEE Method and ACM System are the foundation for changing the perspectives your patients and clients have toward their own potential and achieving the results they want. We must understand that regardless of the programs or services you offer, the patients and clients we are working with may have very different thoughts, ideas and perspectives that need to be addressed.

The difference between a client or patient who achieves success and one who doesn't is most likely due to their own perceptions of what they believe they are capable of and what is possible. You must develop an approach in working with your patients and clients that focuses on their mindset and re-establish this practice over and over again. If you are serious about truly helping your patients and clients achieve extraordinary results, you must adopt a philosophy that is empowering and develops the self-responsibility and positive mindset in your patients and clients. This is what the foundation of The GEE Method embraces.

The Dependency Gap

Ninety-two percent of people suffering from low back pain will leave their doctor's office with a prescription. How is this approach influencing self-reliance, responsibility and independence? The epidemic in opioid drugs over the past decade has illustrated that this approach toward treating pain is not the most effective way and has had tremendous adverse effects on the individual as well as our entire society. Talk about influencing dependency. Although I believe medicine has a place in reducing pain temporarily, it should not be the solution.

Our society has been programmed to wait until pain is present before doing something about it. Once pain has impacted our lives enough, we seek help. The kind of help the majority of people expect is directed toward "what can you do for me to get me out of pain" and as statistics have shown us, results in some type of pill, procedure or product to be the answer.

What I learned through my early career led me to see the health care and fitness industry from a completely different perspective, and I recognized that the paradigm for helping others needed to change. I began seeing more and more people dependent on others for their poor health and fitness. The responsibility was placed on our shoulders, and for me that became a heavy burden.

I realized that the only way I was going to be effective at helping others achieve their health and fitness goals was not reliant on how much more I studied or knew about rehab or physical health. In listening to patients and clients tell me their stories and seeing trends in the health care and fitness industry that cater to the "quick fix" society, I began to understand what needed to be fixed and what needed to be changed.

"What if they just want to walk barefoot?" I ask our clinic doctor regarding one of our patients being fitted for orthotics at the physical therapy clinic where I worked many years ago. The patient would be placed on a treatment table in the prone position (on their stomach) and we would maneuver their ankle into the subtalar neutral position before casting a mold of their foot. Once the cast was set we would remove the mold and determine the most appropriate angles and lift each foot needed for the custom orthotics we were providing patients.

I had spent many years casting molds for custom orthotics and always felt very competent with my skills; however that one day, something just didn't make sense to me. That one question I asked our clinic doctor had challenged the status quo of the practices we, as health care providers, were offering. The doctor's response was one of the first indications that started to make me question if we were really helping people get better or were we the cause of a greater problem?

I am sure you are wondering what the doctor's response was to me after asking him the question about our patient wanting to walk barefoot. I don't recall if he even said anything. I do remember him shrugging his shoulders and shaking his head as if I was wrong in asking such a simple question. That was when I started to question other aspects of what we were providing with patient care. At that moment I knew we were creating dependency for our patients, not hope.

Orthotics were only one of many products we prescribed for patients that were intended to solve their problem. We weren't fixing the reason why this person had poor foot alignment and gait mechanics which caused their pain, we were simply putting a Band-Aid on the problem and creating a dependency on orthotics for this patient. What was this teaching our patients? What other procedures, products and methods were we using that took patients further and further away

64

from self-reliance and personal responsibility? These were the questions I started asking myself with every patient.

We as a society, and specifically the health care and fitness industries, have propagated a culture of quick fixes and dependency on pills, products, procedures and promises to help us with everything that is wrong. We want a solution quickly and with little effort. Our society has become complacent in their health and fitness pursuits and relied heavily on misguided advice and the next "quick fix" product propagated from those viewed as "professionals" in their select fields.

The programs and services we offer should be focused on self-awareness, personal responsibility and an approach that educates and empowers our patients and clients. I began to understand that the current approach toward patient care and personal training was perpetuating a culture of expectations for dependency and quick fixes, with less emphasis on education and empowerment.

Filling the Dependency Gap

The GEE Method philosophy and ACM System were specifically developed to truly support others in achieving personal responsibility. One of the most important questions I ask myself when determining the best approach for each specific client I work with, regardless of their desired goals, is, "Will this empower them to become independent and self-reliant?" Many discussions I have with clients involve advice on products or approaches that they saw or heard about. I help my clients understand what the short-term effects and long-term effects are with the advice I give. I make sure that every client I work with has a deeper level of understanding toward what they are capable of and what their body is capable of, given the right resources.

The ACM System is an objective measure that shows clients what their current body is capable of and what they can achieve through a corrective approach. Many clients may understand that they cannot touch their toes, or have limitations in one of the movement patterns we are assessing, but they may not be aware of how this impacts them in the future. I have always said, *"The signs of a problem are present long before the symptoms occur."* The gentleman who asked me the questions about his hip degeneration acknowledged that at a young age he had many limitations and injuries that were never really addressed, and he is now paying the price for it.

The focus with the ACM System is to identify the movement pattern dysfunctions and postural compensation and use that knowledge to educate your clients on why these problems can or are causing the pain and injury they may be experiencing now or in the future. Remember, unless your client believes they are capable and know it's worth it, they will not have the desire to change or perform any of the corrective exercises you give them. Using the ACM System to assess a client's underlying dysfunctions puts the responsibility in their hands.

As a health care provider and fitness professional, utilizing The GEE Method will give you the knowledge and insights to effectively promote self-responsibility and guide your approach toward establishing a new perspective in the prevention and recovery of injuries and improved performance. The ACM System is your resource that helps you deliver the most effective approach toward helping your patients and clients build the trust and certainty in their own abilities to recover.

The "Focusing on the Symptom not the Problem" Gap

Rx: "Treat for right knee strain"

A referral to physical therapy from a treating physician will indicate a diagnosis specific to the patient's condition with the type, frequency and duration of the rehabilitation indicated. Many times the prescription a treating physician provides the physical therapist is vague. "Treat for right knee strain." The understanding is that physical therapists are competent in their knowledge and understanding of the diagnosis provided and development of the rehabilitation protocol most effective for this patient. Each prescription we were given from the referring doctor was similar to this. The treating physicians knew we were the "experts" in rehabilitation and the trust established allowed us to direct the rehabilitation specific to the doctor's diagnosis for the injured part.

As an athletic trainer, our education was concentrated on the prevention, recognition and recovery of injuries. We are trained to perform specialized joint and muscle testing to determine with some level of certainty the specificity and severity of the injury our athletes sustained. Our approach toward injury recovery and rehabilitation mirrored that of physical therapy. We isolated the injured area and utilized various modalities, stretching techniques and exercises specific to that joint or muscle affected. The focus in health care is on addressing the symptoms or pain and overlooks the contributing factors that led to or compromise the recovery of the injury or pain. In other words, they are not addressing the actual underlying problems.

Nearly every text book I have studied is sectioned off by body part, with an emphasis on the anatomy of the joint, muscle, ligament, nerve and artery involvement and the most common injuries we would expect to encounter for that area. Post-surgery rehabilitation protocols are designed for us to follow, ensuring that we maintain the integrity of the "repaired" tissue during the healing and rehabilitative process. Much research in physical therapy and rehabilitation is focused on the most effective approaches toward recovery efforts of specific joints and muscle activation around the areas of pain and injury.

I equated the time I spent working in physical therapy and sports medicine to that of a well-trained Special Forces sniper. We focused in on the injured area with our high-powered optics and were well-educated on understanding everything we needed to know about that part. We executed our rehabilitation efforts directed at those parts and could rarely go beyond the protocols of the doctor's specific diagnosis. If a patient had shoulder surgery for a repaired rotator cuff, our focus would be on the mitigation of pain and required range of motion and strengthening for that specific shoulder. Even at this level of expertise, focusing on how ankle mobility played a role in shoulder dysfunction was not even a consideration.

The few years I worked in physical therapy were early in my career, and it was exciting to put all the training and education I had learned in college to practice. I admit that I never looked elsewhere in the kinetic chain for underlying dysfunctions or postural compensations. We could see things that didn't look right with a person's posture, but that wasn't our focus nor what the prescription from the doctor allowed us to do. I was excited to use all this knowledge to help people recover from pain and injury, only to find out that I hadn't even scratched the surface in my journey.

The story I described about the patient who was being fitted for custom orthotics was one of the first times I realized that there must be something else we could do to help. The abnormalities in this patient's foot were caused by a greater problem within the kinetic chain.

Although I do not recall the exact circumstances with this patient, I know now, there was a lot more we could have done or worked on that would allow this person to walk barefoot again.

Fast forward ten years from that encounter I had with the treating physician and the lady with orthotics. I was on stage at a doctor's convention discussing this very principle. I asked for a volunteer who had flat feet or collapsing arches. A middle-aged woman stepped up on stage and she was a perfect example of flat feet. Her arches had collapsed, and she mentioned the use of orthotics. The doctors all nodded their heads in agreement of the recommendation for an arch support.

I smiled at the response by the doctors, then asked the lady to tighten her gluteal muscles. With an odd look on her face and with a little coaching she started to learn how to activate her glutes. As she performed this "exercise," I asked the doctors to watch her feet, specifically her arches. The crowd was silent with their mouths dropped open in amazement. As the lady started to squeeze and activate her gluteal muscles the arches of her feet raised up. No artificial support needed, just the right activation of muscles that control joints above and below their location.

The point I was making at this convention was that we need to start looking at why the person's arches were collapsing, not just the fact that they were. More generally, we needed to change the paradigm for treating the problem, not just the symptoms. We needed to change our approach and treatment toward making the results sustainable and reliable.

As I've mentioned, much of my realizations toward the ineffectiveness that I see in rehabilitation, surgery and the approach that health care focuses on came about as a result of my own personal experiences with knee pain and surgeries. At an early age, I was told about the permanent damage I had sustained to my knee, and through my education, I learned that there really wasn't anything that could be done for it. I began to believe what the facts were telling me. I had damaged tissue that does not repair, I had advanced stages of arthritis that was irreversible, and genetically, I was predisposed to tightness and weak cartilage.

The entire focus, since I was ten years old, was on my right knee. Why? Because that is where I had pain and the X-rays and MRIs confirmed the irreversible damage. Seeing these images that the doctors were so happy to show me and explain, also confirmed in my belief that I was broken.

My inability to touch my toes, externally rotated knees and my repetitive ankle sprains were never addressed as part of any rehabilitation efforts or suggestions. As I progressed in my career, eager to find the answers for myself and my patients, I was uncomfortable asking a patient to perform the rehabilitation program I recommended, when I myself couldn't get out of pain. I was experiencing what behaviorists call cognitive dissonance.

I started to question many of the approaches and procedures that I was trained in and knew that with what I was observing through my own personal experience and with the many patients I worked with, it was getting harder for me to continue on the same path. I had finally come to a place where my behaviors were not producing the results I wanted. I had a great reason to improve, but I was missing the pivotal belief that I could actually accomplish it.

It would take me nearly ten more years of searching, studying and perfecting the corrective approach that I discovered to begin to realize that my knee was actually feeling pretty good. The irreversible arthritic damage wasn't causing me problems as predicted and I was living a very active life of training, playing hockey, running and racing motocross and mountain bikes. Those beliefs I had held onto for having irreversible damage were now filled with hope and believing that there was something I could do to help myself.

By only focusing on a patient or client's "symptoms" – their pain – and directing treatment for that specific area, you are only creating a temporary fix. It's easy to take pain away, but to get a patient or client functioning as they were before an injury takes an approach that focuses on helping them believe it's possible and on correcting those underlying conditions that initially predispose them to pain and injury. Focus on the actual problem, the movement pattern and postural compensations, and they will help you truly begin to discover that a symptom is only a sign that something else is wrong. It's your duty to determine what that is.

Filling the "Focusing on the Symptoms Not the Problem" Gap

I will always value the education and experiences I gained working in the health care industry because without it I would not have had the insights to challenge the status quo and begin seeing things from this new perspective. Having the ability to read and decipher medical diagnoses and knowing what it feels like to be told there is nothing that can be done, gives me the leverage to truly help people recover and thrive.

The GEE Method and ACM System is one of the most beneficial and effective assessment systems for identifying and correcting the dysfunctions that cause pain and injury. With every client I work with, I still perform a series of muscle and joint assessments, giving myself and my client a better understanding of what their symptoms are telling us. However, every client will go through the ACM assessment.

My primary goal is to ensure each of my clients understand why movement pattern dysfunctions contribute to, or limit, their ability to recover and what they can do to begin helping themselves improve. The ACM System identifies those underlying dysfunctions and postural compensations and provides the most effective corrective approach, so that clients can begin to see an improvement immediately. Symptoms will come and go while fading over time, but the focus with my clients is to direct their thoughts and actions toward what they have immediate control of, and that is how well they move and function.

I've always felt that a patient should understand their injuries from a cause and effect perspective. It's one thing to diagnose an injury. It's an entirely different perspective to understand what causes tissue stress and damage. The ACM System helps focus your attention on the entire system of functional movement and not specific parts. It teaches you how limited ankle mobility restrictions could be the actual cause of a person's rotator cuff injury. Focusing on the entire kinetic chain is the most effective way to establish the foundation for a patient's full recovery, not just eliminating symptoms or pain.

The Reactive Gap

I still remember the very first sporting event I was responsible for and covering on my own as a brand new athletic trainer. I had spent two years working with the University of New York Buffalo football team and countless hours watching every practice and game from start to end. We stood ready to be called into action if an athlete had been injured – a true practice in patience.

It was a local high school football game, and I was called to cover for a trainer who couldn't make it. I didn't know any of the players and had no idea about their past injury histories or experiences, which added to the stress. I didn't know any of the coaches or their approach with injured athletes. I literally was thrown in the fire that night.

One, Two, Three, Four, Five, Six…. Eleven. After each and every play I counted our team's players as they stood up and made their way back the huddle. I looked for any limping or favoring of body parts to help identify if an athlete had been hurt. I still have no idea who won the game or what the score was. It was the most intense four hours I've ever spent on the sidelines. I was solely responsible for the health and welfare of those kids and took that role very seriously.

As athletic trainers, our focus was on the prevention, recognition and recovery of athletic injuries. The majority of our education and training was directed toward, and our focus was on, the post-injury protocols and procedures. We watched and scanned the field for any fallen players and reacted to their needs as we were trained. In physical therapy we stood ready for every patient that came into our doors to address their pains and injuries. The reactive approach in health care is where one of the greatest problems exists. We wait until there is an injury before doing something about it.

Injuries are hard to predict and an inevitable consequence of participating in an activity or sport at high levels. It would be naïve to say we can prevent all injuries, but I believe many injuries can be minimized tremendously if we focus on what predisposes a person to injury. This goes beyond pre-participation physicals and family history or congenital conditions. I'm talking about biomechanical and postural dysfunctions that strongly contribute to increased risk of pain and injury. These conditions are a result of poor training habits, previous injuries or interacting in the environments that cause poor posture like sitting all the time. We cannot ignore the influence these factors have in predisposing an individual to pain and injury.

Of course, it is important to have trained and competent health care providers to rely on when injuries do occur; however, many of the injuries and chronic pain conditions I've worked with over the years could have been minimized long before the conditions developed. It's one of the biggest reasons I left the traditional role of athletic training and began working on the injury prevention side of the equation. Understanding the mechanism of injuries and identifying underlying conditions that predispose athletes or individuals to injury in the first place should be a stronger focus.

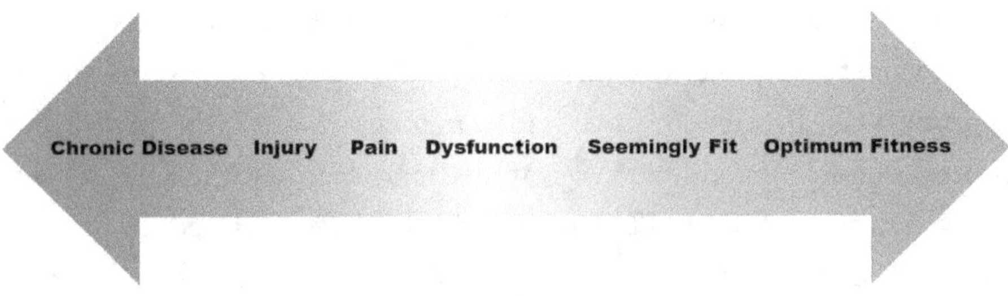

The health spectrum is a great illustration as to the responsibilities of health care providers and fitness professionals. Health care providers are trained more on the left side of the health spectrum, the reactive side. The majority of health care providers wait until a patient comes to them with pain or injury to render care. Fitness professionals work primarily on the right side of the health spectrum, the proactive side. They apply their knowledge and expertise in helping people improve health and fitness. Health care providers focus on the symptoms and treatment of disease while fitness professionals focus on improving the health of their clients

One of the biggest gaps lies between an individual in pain and the seemingly healthy individual, the area of dysfunction. *The signs of pain and injury are present long before the symptoms occur.* Poor postures, limited movement patterns based on joint restrictions and stability motor control are the strongest contributors leading people into pain and injury. These dysfunctions are present in the majority of the population, and addressing these dysfunctions will have the most significant and sustainable results for moving an individual from pain to optimum fitness.

The fitness industry is positioned to be that proactive "injury prevention" resource to those who fall into the dysfunctional category on the health spectrum. Tremendous opportunities are available to fitness professionals who have the knowledge and awareness to identify underlying dysfunctions and postural compensations that predispose individuals to pain and injury. Fitness professionals need to understand the responsibility they have for improving the actual health and fitness of their clients that goes beyond weight loss and getting that sexy summer body.

Too often, I encounter trainers who are not aware of body mechanics, postural compensation and limitations in movement patterns as they ask their clients to perform exercises that reinforce the present dysfunctions. It is the responsibility of the fitness professional to ensure they are leading their clients in the right direction, not back to the doctor's office. Although your clients may appear healthy or fit, it is critical to be aware of any underlying dysfunctions and direct your training toward the correction of those dysfunctions.

A physical therapist, chiropractor or physician will release a patient from care when they have "recovered" from the injury or the pain they were experiencing. Unfortunately, in many cases, patients are released from care due to lack of insurance reimbursement and only received a minimal amount of therapy visits. Patients are left to their own accord with very little guidance or direction in self-care. Remember, the health care industry is built on dependency, not self-responsibility.

Even patients released from a health care provider, who no longer have pain, may still have significant dysfunction related to their posture, movement pattern restriction and limitations. The role of most health care providers is to "fix" the pain, not the dysfunction that may have contributed to the symptom. Patients may recover from pain and injury temporarily from the treatment of the health care providers, but many times, the symptoms return or manifest elsewhere.

The majority of individuals who seek the guidance of personal trainers have aches, pains, previous injuries or are released from the care of a health care provider for various reasons. Many people are worried and intimidated about beginning to exercise because of the previous injuries and pain they may still have. The fitness professional must have a deeper understanding of the role they play in the health care and fitness spectrum to ensure they are making the right decisions for their client's benefit.

The fitness professional should be proactively addressing underlying postural conditions and movement pattern dysfunctions that strongly contribute to pain and injury. Regardless of a client's goals in the gym, a fitness professional has the ability to impact the lives of the clients tremendously if they approach the training from the perspective of injury prevention and develop the knowledge and skills to be effective at correcting dysfunction first.

I've learned many lessons toward effective injury prevention approaches working in the field of ergonomics. The goal with ergonomics is to "engineer out the risk." What this means is, if there is an object in the center of the floor, for example, I can teach you how to walk around it so you don't trip, or I can remove the object and you will never have to worry about tripping. A strong ergonomic program encompasses a proactive approach ensuring that job tasks, procedures, equipment and tools are designed, selected and built to minimize risk. We don't wait until an injury occurs before we say, "Oh, I guess we should have moved that object."

I was fortunate to have the opportunity to work in ergonomics and field test the principles of the GEE Method and ACM System with employees. The programs and services I provide corporations are the same programs and services I deliver in the GEE Method and ACM Program to the health care providers and fitness professionals. Many companies are starting to understand the concept of "an ounce of prevention is worth a pound of cure." As health care providers and fitness professionals, we, too, should embrace this advice in working with our patients and clients.

One of the more concerning issues that I have experienced in working with thousands of clients over the years is the way they account for their injuries. Many people develop low back pain, neck pain, shoulder pain or knee pain as a result of doing nothing out of the ordinary. "I must have slept wrong," "I was just bending over to tie my shoes," "I was kneeling down to pick up something on the floor" or "I was just reaching to grab a book."

These are the seemingly healthy individuals who appear to be doing fine and aren't aware of or having any health concerns, dysfunctions. They are not experiencing levels of pain or discomfort that worry them. They go about their day-to-day tasks and exercise as if everything is fine, until "BAM" – one day they experience a sudden sharp pain in their neck, back, shoulder or knee. This results in blaming the task or exercise for the injury and not the underlying dysfunction that actually caused it.

That person now has a "symptom" and goes to the doctor or chiropractor to find out what is wrong. They are treated for their specific pain. They may be told to stop running or only sleep a certain way, because this is what causes their pain. In reality what caused their injury is the underlying dysfunction that led to postural compensation and misuse of the affected muscle or joint. *The signs of an injury are present long before the symptoms occur* and the reactive model for injury recovery can be shortened and more effective if we started to understand how to identify and correct the actual problem

Filling the Reactive Gap

Many years ago, I remember reading an article in the **San Diego Tribune**. Yes, a newspaper! It was during the spring, a time when everyone was starting to get ready for swimsuit season. The article was about spring cleaning for our bodies and how to protect ourselves from getting injured. The author pointed out many movements that they deemed risky and that should be avoided. They used examples like, "If you are not a rooster, then you shouldn't tilt your neck back", "If you are not a baseball catcher, you shouldn't do a deep squat," and various other examples that I don't specifically remember. What I do remember is the entire article was explaining to readers that we should avoid all sorts of movements that will cause pain and damage to our body.

Although the author's intention was to offer a "proactive" approach to helping people avoid getting injured, the suggestion to avoid activities and movements that our body is actually designed to perform only perpetuates the fears people have about physical activity. Our bodies were designed for all kinds of movement, and to limit movement due to fear, pain or limitation leads to a sedentary lifestyle.

The authors of an article from The Cooper Institute titled, "*The Effect of Physical Inactivity and Obesity on Morbidity and Mortality: Current Evidence and Research Issues.*" (Blair, SN and Brodney, S, Med Sci Sports Exerc. 1999 Nov. 31(11 Suppl): S646-62), concluded that regular physical activity clearly attenuates many of the health risks associated with being overweight or obese:

- Physical activity appears to not only attenuate the health risks of overweight and obesity, but active obese individuals actually have lower morbidity and mortality than normal weight individuals who are sedentary.

- Inactivity and low cardiorespiratory fitness are as important as overweight and obesity as mortality predictors.

I would hope as health care providers and fitness professionals we agree that we need to move. Suggesting that movement should be minimized and limited is not being proactive, it's being irresponsible. As health care and fitness professionals, it is our job to understand the design of the human body, its capabilities and how to best improve the lives of our patients and clients without restricting or limiting movement. The proactive approach may challenge you to begin looking at your current methods, services and procedures differently, but will provide the greatest benefit to your patients and clients.

The ACM System is one of the most effective "proactive" approaches toward identifying and correcting the underlying movement pattern dysfunctions and postural compensations your patients and clients have. The ACM Corrective Exercise Therapy Specialist certification course provides you with the knowledge to identify those underlying dysfunctions and a proven method for correcting the problems before another person has to suffer from pain.

Being proactive toward injury prevention and improving physical performance should be the ultimate goal for the health care and fitness industries. Establishing yourself as the expert in corrective exercise therapy and injury prevention only takes a change in your perspective from reactive to proactive. Learning the ACM System will ensure you have the knowledge, resources and expertise to establish yourself as a leader in an industry desperate for a proactive approach.

The "Focusing on the Parts" Gap

"You are the reason my weight lifting bar got bent?"

My first experiences in weight lifting, and what I would later understand to be functional training, came at the age of ten, during a trip to New Jersey to visit my aunt, uncle and cousins. My cousin, Keir, was a Mr. Teen bodybuilder, and being six years older than me, he really wasn't interested in showing me the ropes, or having me tag along with him to the gym. In the few interchanges I had with him that weekend, I noticed he had a weight lifting bar in his room with a few steel plates on it. Inspired by his physique and how he talked about bodybuilding, I thought I'd give it a try when no one was looking. We had the car packed and everyone was saying goodbye. As you may imagine, the patience of a ten-year-old boy was short, and the goodbye process was a long, drawn out event, because we only saw them a few times a year. While everyone was embraced in hugs and kisses, I ran into his room eager to stake my claim next to his bodybuilding titles.

I grabbed that bar and heaved it over my head quickly, amazed at my freakish strength, only to realize it was still going. Over my head the bar soared and landed on the floor with a huge bang. I didn't even turn to look at what had happened. I ran out the door saying goodbye to everyone on the way to the car. Years later, during Christmas with the entire family, stories about the old days came up, and I finally came clean. My cousin finally found out how his weight bar became bent.

A few years following the bent bar incident, I started working out in a real gym. I was 12 years old and this gym was a small mom and pop place near my house. I went every day after school with a handwritten workout plan my cousin had developed for me. He said it was what he did to get so big and all I would need. I followed it to the letter.

Each body part laid out with the exact number of sets and reps required to grow muscle. Back then, there were no fancy machines and only a few funny looking bars that I had no idea what to do with. He told me to stick to the basics, so if you ever went to another gym and they didn't have the specific machine or fancy bar, you wouldn't be thrown off.

By the age of 16, bodybuilding had consumed me, and I competed in my first contest and took 2nd. The year before was when I tore my meniscus in gym class and had to sit out the entire following season of football. I really didn't care because lifting had become my passion. I was seeing the results, but something interesting started to happen to me. I became more interested in why my muscles were growing. What was it about lifting weight that caused our muscles to grow?

There were only a few muscle magazines at the time that featured freakishly huge professional bodybuilders and their secret workouts for each body part. My first introduction to human anatomy came from the glossy pages of those muscle magazines, and I would take each exercise illustrated and try to learn which muscle was working and why they responded the way they did. The only advice we received was from other "fitness" enthusiasts and those magazines. We didn't have

THE KEIR WAY TO GETTING BIG AND STRONG

MONDAY (CHEST + BACK)
FLAT BENCH — 5 SETS — 4-8 REPS
INCLINE BENCH — 3 SETS — 4-8 REPS
BENT OVER ROWS — 5 SETS — 4-8 REPS
LAT PULLDOWNS — 3 SETS — 4-10 REPS

WEDNESDAY (SHOULDERS, ARMS)
STANDING MILITARY PRESS — 5 SETS — 4-8 REPS
UPRIGHT ROWS — 3 SETS — 6-10 REPS
DIPS — 5 SETS — 4-8 REPS
PUSHDOWNS — 3 SETS — 4-8 REPS
STANDING LONG BAR CURL — 5 SETS — 4-8 REPS
STANDING HAMMER CURLS — 3 SETS — 6-10 REPS

FRIDAY (LEGS)
SQUATS — 5 SETS — 4-8 REPS
LEG PRESS — 3 SETS — 4-8 REPS
LEG CURLS — 3 SETS — 6-10 REPS
STANDING CALF RAISES — 5 SETS — 6-12 REPS

ALL MUST BE DONE SUPER STRICT!
— NO FORCED REPS
— ONLY HELP ON LAST REP
— EAT EVERYTHING IN SIGHT

exercise science and kinesiology majors as personal trainers and if you looked good, we listened. We learned from the streets, so to speak.

By the time I was 18 and facing the impending doom of my second knee surgery, my interest in bodybuilding was focused more on the science of bodybuilding. I always enjoyed lifting heavy weights, but it was the medical side of the equation that really interested me most. I started my first personal training job at a local gym and thrived on teaching clients about fitness. Early in my professional career in fitness, I remember thinking that all it takes to be a personal trainer was to have a nice physique, look like you know what you are doing, and people would listen to you. I never felt comfortable with that premise, which is why I studied as much as I could with the limited resources available to us at the time.

I became a master at training parts. I had my Chest and Triceps day, Back and Biceps day and my Legs and Shoulder days. It's how everyone trained back then, and I experimented with all kinds of different exercises to get the best isolation and size. With my growing knowledge in exercise science, the gym became my research and development department. I would manipulate sets, reps, volume and intensity to get the most effective gains for each part I trained.

The fitness industry focuses on exercise in a similar way to the health care industry's focus on the treatment of injuries and pain. Each workout and program is designed to isolate and emphasize individual body parts. The best exercise for your (insert body part here) can be found in every YouTube video and fitness magazine out there and provides misleading and misguided advice for the unsuspecting public. The emphasis on training body parts is still ingrained in the gym culture and perceptions of those who dream of getting those big muscles and toned bodies. The emergence of the functional training trend, which I will discuss in the next "GAP" section, has shifted some of the focus away from the parts, but it's still there as the foundation to weight training and fitness for many personal trainers.

In the second section of this book, you will learn in more detail about corrective exercise and the influence everything we do has on the body's functional capabilities. For now, it is critical to understand that we can never isolate one muscle group or body part. Even the most specific machines that are used in every health club and gym or the exercises that focus on a specific body part are still influenced by and influencing the rest of the muscular system. This is the greatest mistake most health care providers and fitness professionals make. They neglect to understand what is happening with the entire system and how to identify and correct dysfunctions. Focusing on individual parts only reinforces what is already wrong.

——— Filling the "Focusing on the Parts" Gap ———

"I need to start doing what you are doing. How did you survive that crash, again?" - Friend

Racing motocross was an experience of the greatest highs and lowest lows. There was nothing that can compare to jumping through the air, sometimes over 90 feet, with no safety net or certainty that you were going to make it. Along with the thrill of it all came the agony of defeat. Not only losing, but crashing. And we crashed a lot; it was just part of that sport.

Much of my training and ambition to be in top physical condition was not to perform better or to win, but to survive the crashes we experienced. I had dislocated my shoulder in one race at the beginning of the season in March. Five months after surgery and rehab, I got back on the track to get the rust off and begin preparing to race again. This picture happened to be that day when I returned back on the track. A friend had been taking pictures of my buddy and me pushing each other's limits throughout the day. He happened to catch this big crash of mine as it unfolded. I hit the ground at about 30 miles per hour after negotiating a jump the wrong way. The sequence of photos shows the end result. I hit the ground pretty hard, and my day of riding was over because my handle bars were bent, but I was okay. The shoulder I had spent five months rehabbing is the same shoulder that I landed on.

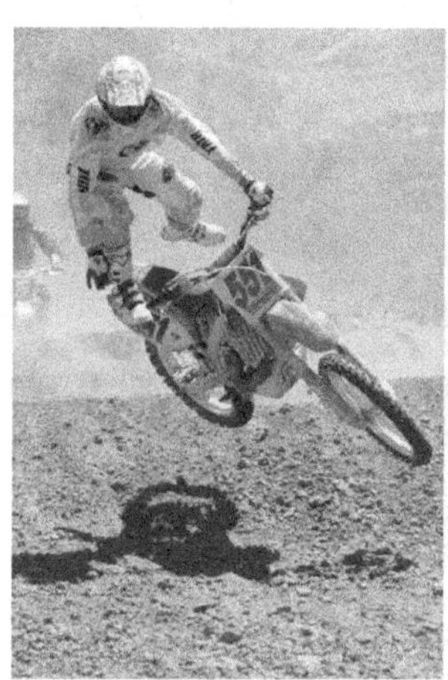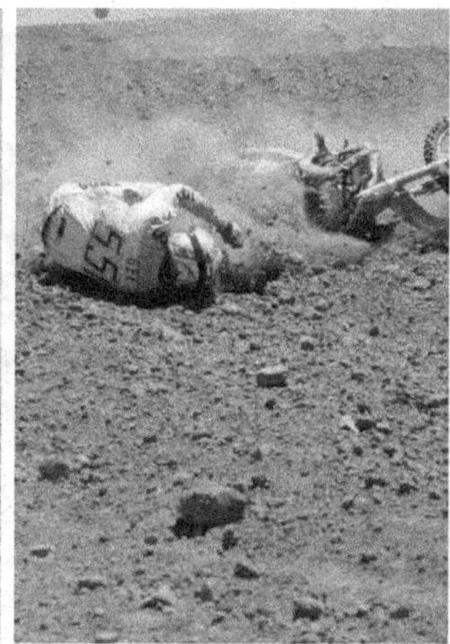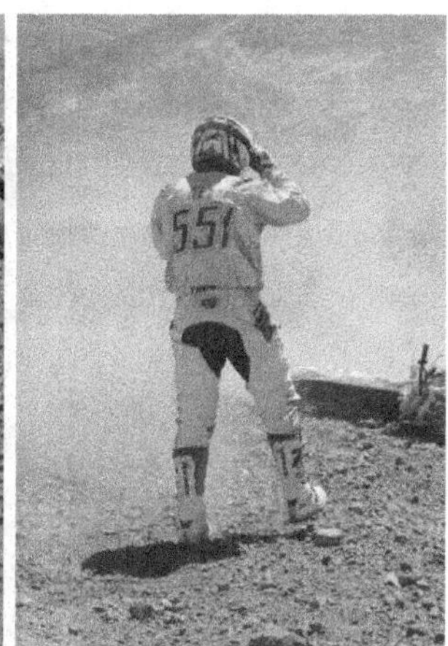

When I returned to the trucks, my friends were already packing up frantically, assuming they were going to have to get me to the hospital ASAP. I told them I was fine and just a little scratched up. My friend was shocked, because he was the one right behind me watching it happen. He said, "Gee (that's what everyone calls me), I don't know what you are doing for training, but I need to start doing it, too."

I learned through a lot of injuries and pain early in my athletic endeavors that lifting weights through isolating muscle groups made me bigger and stronger but didn't make me a better athlete or help me in preventing possible injuries. In fact, what I began to learn during my journey was that the lifting I was doing, which was predominately training parts, was actually perpetuating many of the nagging injuries and pain I experienced, especially my knees. The methods of "fitness" I had surrounded myself with in the gyms was actually predisposing me to injuries with everything I was doing. I just hadn't put the pieces of the puzzle together yet.

Like many of you who train this way, I feel like I could run through a brick wall. As I've gotten older, I just have to back up a little further now. (That was a joke – or was it?) Training like this makes us feel strong and invincible; however we all have a brick wall. That brick wall for me was my knee pain, and what I discovered later to be the dysfunctional movement patterns I was strengthening as I trained my parts. Most of us simply try to build a stronger, more resilient body because the brick wall seems to get thicker and taller. That brick wall we all have becomes tougher to navigate over time, not because we are getting older, but because the longer we train parts, the greater the dysfunctions will be reinforced. The deeper those underlying movement pattern dysfunctions are, the higher and thicker that brick wall becomes.

I often use the analogy of a person driving around with their emergency brake on. After a while they notice the car isn't running like it used to, so they take it to the auto mechanic. This would be the equivalent of a person coming to you because they know their body needs help. The auto mechanic can put a bigger motor in the car, more efficient gas, all of which will make the car run stronger, or he can just reach in and take the emergency brake off. Identify why the car isn't running well and identify why the body isn't running well before just assuming it needs a stronger motor or muscle.

It wasn't easy to do. I had spent my entire life in the gym and perfected my "parts" game. The gym and what I knew was my comfort zone, yet as my knees improved and my body felt better, I knew this new form of training was the answer. I was correcting the dysfunctions that held me back from moving, repairing and performing at a higher level. I was developing an entirely different type of strength and function that was necessary to withstand the crashes and recover from the inevitable injuries I had while racing. I didn't have to break through that brick wall any more. I simply took the emergency brakes off. Most of your patients and clients are running around with an emergency brake on and don't even realize it.

The ACM System is the foundation that will benefit all prevention, rehabilitation and training programs. Learning how to identify the most underlying movement pattern dysfunctions and postural compensations (those emergency brakes) with a proven corrective approach is the most beneficial way to unlock the body's greatest potential. The ACM System was developed to augment what most health care providers and fitness professionals are currently offering. The added value of identifying and correcting the underlying dysfunctions and postural compensations is necessary to ensure you are providing the most beneficial and sustainable results for your patients and clients.

The HIIT Training and Functional Training Gap

The concept of functional training is nothing new. We have used a form of functional training in the rehabilitation setting for years. The focus with Occupational Therapists, Physical Therapists and Athletic Trainers is to utilize functional training to restore movement disorders with their patients. Functional training's true conception was to establish or re-establish an individual's ability to perform the activities of daily life, ADLs.

Physical therapists first started using functional training to help a patient bridge the gap between recovering from an injury or surgery and returning them back to "functioning" in the activities, sports or tasks of their daily life. Unfortunately, due to insurance reimbursements, limited therapy visits and an emphasis on getting people out of pain quickly, the use of functional training in the rehab setting is very limited.

What is functional training? It depends on who you are asking. The overall concept is that exercise or training is designed for whole body movements, not isolation, as was traditional in the fitness industry; moving many joints through full ranges of motion and through all three planes of motion, as opposed to the single plane of motion most gym workout machines and equipment facilitate. Functional training mimics the actions one must perform through normal daily activities and sports.

Unilateral movement patterns – like a single leg lunge – that include the rotational lifting or chopping component of the upper extremity is a more functional movement pattern than a squat. The squat is a more functional movement pattern than the leg press. The leg press is a more functional movement pattern than the leg extension machine.

These examples illustrate that the less reliant on machines and more complex the movement pattern is, the more functional the movement can be considered to be.

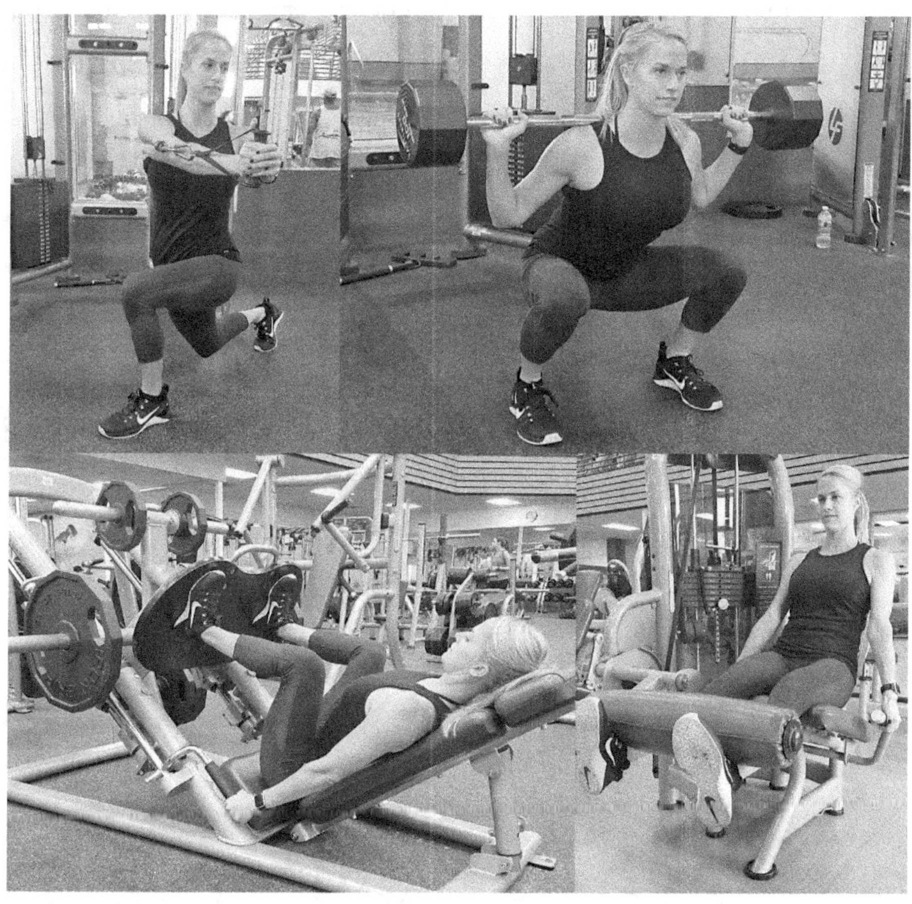

Utilizing full body movements through multiple planes of motion that require the mobility and stability of the entire body would be a relatively strong statement for defining functional training. By performing exercises this way, the body must be getting more functional, right? This is where the greatest misconceptions and misguided information are amongst the fitness community.

One of the first mass "functional training" gyms was introduced to the public in 2000. Greg Glassman, the founder of CrossFit, developed this unique workout and gym experience that was truly different than what was available at the time, and people started to migrate from the large corporate gyms to this specialized niche workout regimen.

> *CrossFit is a strength and conditioning program consisting mainly of a mix of aerobic exercise, calisthenics (body weight exercises), and Olympic weightlifting. CrossFit, Inc. describes its strength and conditioning program as "constantly varied functional movements executed at high intensity across broad time and modal domains," with the stated goal of improving fitness, which it defines as "work capacity across broad time and modal domains."*
>
> *CrossFit gyms use equipment from multiple disciplines, including barbells, dumbbells, gymnastics rings, pull-up bars, jump ropes, kettlebells, medicine balls, plyo boxes, resistance bands, rowing machines, and various mats. CrossFit is focused on "constantly varied, high-intensity, functional movement," drawing on categories and exercises such as these: calisthenics, Olympic-style weightlifting, powerlifting, Strongman-type events, plyometric, body weight exercises, indoor rowing, and aerobic exercise, running, and swimming.*
>
> *"CrossFit is not a specialized fitness program, but a deliberate attempt to optimize physical competence in each of 10 recognized fitness domains," says founder Greg Glassman in the Foundations document. Those domains are: cardiovascular and respiratory endurance, stamina, strength, flexibility, power, speed, coordination, agility, balance, and accuracy.*
>
> https://en.wikipedia.org/wiki/CrossFit

Around the time CrossFit was changing how people viewed workouts, a new exercise concept called HIIT Training, High Intensity Interval Training, started to become popular. HIIT is a workout that involves high intensity exercise bouts for short periods of time, followed by a lower intensity exercise repeated until exhaustion. This type of training has been shown to increase athletic conditioning and fat loss. This new concept was added to the functional training programs and a whole new fitness trend was started.

Performing high intensity "functional" exercises continuously until exhaustion meant that you could complete a workout in less time and feel like you spent hours training. The belief that because you were doing primarily body weight exercises, through large ranges and multiple planes of motion, you were getting in shape and "functional." Many of the hybrid programs out there now use Olympic-style lifting with various bands, straps and devices to increase the demands of mobility and stability through the workout. These gyms and workouts are popping up everywhere and influencing the general public's perception of what functional training is.

"If you are not functional to start with, functional training will not make you functional – it will get you hurt."

-MICHAEL GEE

During high intensity exercises, you are asking for many joints and muscle systems to work together to accomplish the movement or exercise. The coordinated efforts of every joint and muscle group needs to be precise, or your body will compensate and find the path of least resistance. Asking a person to jump onto a box or off a box as part of a functional training program doesn't ensure they are capable of the ankle and hip mobility, along with the torso stability required to perform this movement effectively. If you continue to ask someone to perform high intensity movements without correcting underlying dysfunctions, you are only increasing the risk of injury to that person.

"Look at this, Mike, these are the same types of exercises you have had us doing for years," said my friend when he brought an article to me one day about the person who founded CrossFit. At first, it was exciting to hear that the concepts of functional training had started being introduced in the fitness industry for the general public to benefit from. Through my journey in discovering how to help myself with the knee pain I experienced my entire life, I had moved away from the gyms and fitness community and was performing functional exercises on my own, long before it was a trend.

When I run my functional boot camp classes, the focus is on identifying any underlying dysfunctions with my clients and correcting them with specific exercise programs and sequences as part of the entire workout, paying close attention to the quality of work, not the quantity my clients performed. If I notice a client performing a squat or lunge with faulty or dysfunctional patterns, I will modify the exercise to ensure they are working at the appropriate level their body can handle. I know too well, if I pushed a client whose knees were buckling inward during a squat, or who had ankle mobility restrictions and was trying to perform a box jump, I was only reinforcing what their body already knew to do. They would get hurt and I would be out of business quickly.

I have always said, "You can make a person sprint up a hill until they throw up, but it doesn't mean they got a great workout." The signs of a great workout are that you have improved and reinforced correct movement patterns and function, not just fatigued muscles and made a person breathe hard and sweat. The challenge with performing high intensity exercise is that a person may not have the ability to perform the movement correctly. Their physical capabilities are at a lower threshold. A person can get more out of a lower threshold movement or exercise because you are focusing on their true weaknesses and dysfunctions. Once corrected, the person can move to a higher-level threshold with more certainty and safety.

As functional training began to emerge in the fitness industry, I started paying a little more attention to the fitness professionals who were influencing this movement. In a short period of time, I discovered that the concept of "functional training" that I had employed for myself and my clients was far different than what the fitness industry had adopted. The focus seemed to cater to the clients who wanted a shorter workout and still feel like they spent hours at the gym. Throw in some "functional" exercises and you can call it "functional training".

The perception the general public has toward functional training is far from what functional really was intended for and is. Unfortunately, as seemingly healthy individuals begin to be seduced into this new promising exercise program, injuries will begin to happen. If you ask many who joined the CrossFit programs in the early years, they will tell you they were either injured or they know people who did get injuries from that type of training. As other gyms and trainers begin to market their functional training programs, more unsuspecting individuals will dive in. They have been told they need to strengthen their core and functional training will provide what they need. When these people get injured, where do they turn?

If you tell a person who was injured that they need to strengthen their core after being injured strengthening their core, what do you think their response will be? There are many programs and exercises of the week that promise to improve core strength and function. I've witnessed many clients who partake in these "only 5 exercises to a stronger core" programs. In watching them perform the high-level movements, the dysfunctions that are present only get reinforced.

One of the more memorable experiences I had related to the "core strengthening" was a group of gentlemen who committed to holding each other accountable for doing one specific core exercise every day. As a group, they would get together at the same time and one of them would time their front planks. Their goal was to hold the front plank for three minutes and they worked at this each day. They told me that one of the men found a website that said all you need to do is a front plank for the most effective core exercise. These guys were convinced. I'm sure the person promoting this had a six-pack of chiseled abs and was obviously convincing. In watching them perform the movement, none of them looked the same. Each gentleman was doing the front plank a little different than the others. One guy's hips were tucked under and his upper back was completely rounded. Another guy's hips were not level – yes, one hip was higher than the other. One guy's shoulder was pulled up toward his ears like he was doing shrugs. How is this one core exercise influencing core strength if none of them were even doing it correctly?

Each of them understood how to do the exercise; however, what their brain knew and what their body was capable of were not the same. As I pointed out the dysfunctions and compensated strengths, they were more inclined to step back from the higher-level exercise and do a few exercises that I gave them, specific to their actual dys-functions. Who cares if you can hold a front plank for three minutes if you can't even touch your toes or effectively bend over to pick up your child without hurting your back? Core strengthening is much more complex than the front plank remedy.

I'm not saying the front plank is bad. I'm not saying any functional or core exercise is bad. It's only bad if it's not performed correctly, and it is the trainer's responsibility to understand what dysfunction and compensation is to most effectively benefit their clients. The fitness industry has a tremendous opportunity and responsibility to provide the most effective approach to improving the health and fitness of the general public, both physically and mentally. Functional training, performed appropriately with an emphasis on actually identifying and correcting movement pattern dysfunction and postural compensation, is the most beneficial way to ensure the functional training trend is moving in the right direction, all pun intended!

Filling the HIIT Training and Functional Training Gap

"How did you know I have a right hip problem?"

– ANONYMOUS

I heard about a new gym that had opened near my house and the name intrigued me. It was a pure functional training gym and the information on their website drew me in. Everything they spoke about was very enticing and I knew I had to check it out. When I arrived at the gym, they were halfway through one of the group classes they offered, so I waited on the side to speak to the owner/trainer.

I observed the circuit of functional exercises each member was performing – 45 seconds at one station and then they would move to the next station. This went on for the full 45 minutes with a 20–to-30 second rest period in the middle. Each exercise emphasized full body movements, some specialized equipment like pullups and medicine ball throws, but overall, I would say it was a pretty complete HIIT training workout and far from a "functional" workout.

When the class ended, the owner/trainer came up to me with a huge smile on her face and welcomed me to her club. I explained that I was excited to learn that a true functional training gym had opened, and I was there to observe. I told her about my experience in corrective exercise and sports medicine and then explained what the ACM program was all about. I told her about her right hip issue she had, which I observed while she was performing all of the functional training exercises. Her mouth dropped and asked, "How did you know I had a right hip problem?"

I had only begun putting the ACM certification course together, and leaving that workout, I knew that this program was more necessary now than ever. As a way to explain how the ACM program could benefit her gym and members, I asked the owner a very compelling question, "What happens when one of your members gets injured? Do you think they are coming back to a functional training gym again, needless to say your gym?"

I admire the innovation with exercise that I've seen in the fitness industry, moving from single plane, isolated exercises like the bench press to variations of pushups that emphasize multi-plane movement patterns of the entire body. Each of these exercises has tremendous value if performed correctly with the understanding of true function and the awareness to identify faulty patterns and dysfunction. The more progressive, demanding and "functional" an exercise and movement pattern is, the more important it is to address and correct the underlying dysfunctions that will be reinforced due to the compensation.

The foundation to function is the most important aspect to any injury prevention, recovery and improved performance agenda.

The ACM System of movement pattern assessments and corrective exercise therapy is the foundation to addressing these underlying dysfunctions to ensure you are building a solid base for your patients and clients to work from. Without a strong foundation, all you are doing is reinforcing the problems, regardless of how functional you may think the workout is. ACM helps you identify those underlying conditions and gives you the tools and resources to establish yourself as a corrective exercise specialist and a true functional training expert.

The Pride and Ego Gap

"I know that" are the three worst words in the English language.

The world is filled with all kinds of things that you certainly know. There are other things in the world that you know you don't know, like knowing there is a different language, but you don't speak it. Then there are things out there that we don't know we don't know. This area is much larger than the other two, and if you are open and willing to accept that learning is a continuous process there is so much more to discover. By saying, "I know that," you are shutting off any possibility to learn and grow. Staying in your comfort zone may seem safe but it's not where you are able to make the greatest differences in your life with others.

My professional career started at The University of New York at Buffalo. The athletic training staff consisted of the head trainer, two assistant trainers and about ten student trainers. As the head student trainer my senior year, I was a big fish in a small pond. I was developing the competency and confidence to grow in this field. As I began expanding my network and career path in physical therapy and graduate school, I was exposed to very experienced and knowledgeable therapists and trainers. Each step of my career path, I worked toward establishing my expertise in the discipline in which I was working.

What we did on the sports field as athletic trainers was very different from what we did in the clinical setting for physical therapy. Although I was confident in my basic understanding of injury recognition and recovery, I quickly realized that my level of education, knowledge and experience was only the beginning. When I started working in Ergonomics, I had to learn an entirely new vocabulary and professional discipline. Each time I made the decision to work outside my comfort zone, I had to step my pride and ego back to allow myself the opportunity to grow and learn.

When I was first introduced to the corrective exercise field as part of my journey to find the answers I had been looking for, it provoked my "fight or flight" response. My experience and certainty that I had developed in the sports medicine field was now being questioned and challenged. I had read a book that talked about posture and how correcting faulty posture was the way to recover from injuries. This made sense in theory; we learned a little about posture analysis in college, but never really focused on the corrective aspects for injury prevention and recovery, at least not at the scale that this book was talking about.

I spent almost seven years learning the skills and concepts of injury recognition and recovery, and was developing the experience, confidence and certainty that I needed to establish myself in this career. When I began studying corrective exercise therapy, I realized quickly that I had a lot more to learn. The ideas related to underlying conditions and how to identify and correct these problems made too much sense. I knew that this was the right path, even though it was going to take me way outside of my comfort zone, and it would take time for me to develop the level of expertise I had already achieved – the theory was something I couldn't ignore.

Turning down a position with a professional sports team was a significant decision that I had to make early in my career. My ego and pride would have to be put aside as I learned corrective exercise therapy. I believed that the concepts of identifying dysfunction and the results I was seeing with corrective exercise were the most beneficial way of preventing and recovering from injuries. My decision wasn't easy and corrective exercise therapy would take time to adapt into the health care and fitness industries, but I saw the results and knew it was the path I needed to pursue.

One of the hardest things for most people to do is step outside of their comfort zones. As professionals in health care and fitness, that comfort zone is established with a higher level of education, experience and certainty in the methods and services you offer. We build the necessary levels of confidence and credibility in our chosen professions, which also comes with the responsibility to our patients and clients to always be growing and exploring new opportunities for their benefit.

> *"Do what is right, not what is easy nor what is popular."*
>
> – ROY T. BENNETT

As health care and fitness professionals, our responsibility is to act as fiduciaries, always providing what is most beneficial to our patients and clients. Their best interest must be our first priority and the programs and services we offer should not be inhibited or restricted by what we believe is best for our egos and pride. I have met many therapists and trainers who are open to learning and expanding their levels of knowledge and expertise; however, the health care and fitness industry is also crippled by egos and pride – those who are unwilling to step outside their comfort zones and allow for new opportunities of growth and development.

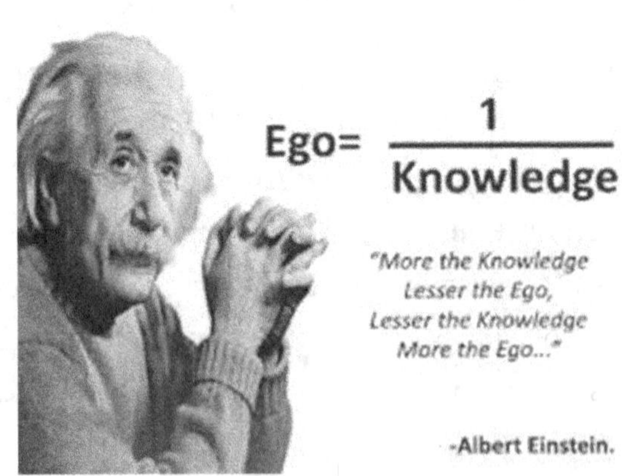

I have had many mentors throughout my career and continue to seek knowledge and understanding as part of my ever-continuing education. Beyond the CEU requirements of our licenses and certifications, I believe it is necessary to challenge ourselves and be open to new paths and directions far outside our comfort zones. The most successful and acclaimed professional in health care and fitness have mentors who encourage them to broaden their skills, knowledge and experience. Setting aside our egos, pride and established credentials can be challenging, but necessary to influence an industry for the greater good.

The fitness industry is constantly evolving and our knowledge of exercise physiology, kinesiology and how to produce the most effective results has never been more researched and documented. Those fitness professionals who have dedicated their careers toward researching, learning and understanding human performance are helping move the fitness industry forward with some resistance, no pun intended.

The fitness industry is a mixture of well-educated professionals, as well as "fitness enthusiasts." The well-educated professionals either pursue an exercise science or kinesiology degree in college or have taken the responsibility to learn hands-on with a passion for helping others achieve greater health and fitness goals. Regardless of the path taken, those well-educated fitness professionals value the science and wonder of the human body and embody what the fitness industry truly needs to make an impact on the overall health of the general public. Unfortunately, the fitness industry is congested with fitness enthusiasts who have achieved high levels of fitness for themselves and feel this is what qualifies them to train others. This is where a tremendous gap lies.

The entry-level requirements to become a "personal trainer" are minimal. Many gyms and health clubs will have their own entry level certification program or internship or require an entry-level certification from an accrediting agency like NASM, The National Academy of Sports Medicine, for example. There are many organizations one can get their personal training certification credentials from and each has value as entry-level knowledge. You only need to be 18 years old and have a high school diploma or GED equivalent in most cases.

The median salaries for personal trainers is around $56,000, and many who graduate with degrees in exercise science or kinesiology move on to higher levels of education or transition into a higher-growth field. The majority of personal trainers embark on this path because of their personal interests in fitness and the simplicity of obtaining the entry-level credentials. Some go on to become well-educated and have a positive influence in the industry, while many simply maintain their entry-level status.

The perspective of the general public toward the fitness industry is that we are highly-educated health professionals. Our influence toward helping individuals achieve health and fitness goals also comes with great responsibility. This responsibility goes beyond a slimmer waist and bigger muscles as is the focus of much of the fitness industry promotion. As a professional in the fitness industry, it is critical that you understand the influence you have on the general public and the perception of the industry.

The realities of the fitness industry are that many personal trainers are simply fitness enthusiasts who are underqualified to work with the majority of the general public. The false assumption that clients are coming to us seemingly healthy is one of the greatest mistakes a personal trainer can make. This is what separates those who are fitness enthusiasts from the ones who can truly have an impact on the health and safety of their clients.

Clients are coming to you for your expertise in health and fitness. They assume you have the qualifications to address their concerns about general health, previous injuries or aches and pains they may be currently experiencing. Believe me, most of your clients have previous injuries or aches and pains that they believe "getting into better shape" will address. They are with you because they don't know what to do or they don't want to get hurt. It is your responsibility to have those qualifications and not ignore potential risk factors that can predispose your clients to further injury.

Those risk factors I'm speaking about are not related to heart rate, blood pressure and the previous medical history intake. I'm speaking of the underlying movement pattern dysfunctions and postural compensations that contribute to increased risk of pain and injury. I witness too many trainers who demonstrate to the best of their ability how to perform a particular exercise, only to watch their clients struggling. Not struggling with the selected weight or intensity level, but struggling with their inability to stabilize the load of their body or compensate due to the demand of the exercise. To a trained and educated professional, these compensated movement patterns and postural dysfunctions stand out like a sore thumb. To the fitness enthusiast, they write down the number of sets, reps and weights and move on.

A well-trained fitness professional would have the knowledge and experience to understand that each client needs to be performing at their body's capability. The exercise program that was developed for them would focus on the quality of the movement, not the number of reps, sets and weight. Having the knowledge to recognize and correct damaging dysfunctions is what separates the great trainers from the fitness enthusiasts.

Filling the Pride and Ego Gap

For a moment, I want you to reflect on the philosophy and approach you are currently taking with your clients and patients. If you struggle with understanding what your philosophy is or what the final outcome your programs and services truly offer, it's time to establish for yourself what that looks like. Too often we get stuck in the day-to-day procedures of what we are already great at and have a hard time seeing it from the third-party perspective. One of the greatest questions I always ask myself is, "Would I send my loved one to someone like me?" It helps me keep a perspective for what influence I am having on my clients and helps me stay on the path I've established for myself.

The GEE Method and ACM System was developed to augment, and in many cases, replace the current philosophy and approach you are taking. Yes, this may mean that you will have to take a step back and evaluate how effective your current approach is at treating the entire person, not just their symptoms or their perspective on what health and fitness is. Most of us have entered the health care and fitness professions to make a difference, and that difference needs to be established in how you conduct yourself and the programs and services you offer. What are your limits and deal breakers when it comes to treating and working with your clients and patients? What is your direction and purpose overall? Your philosophy is your "north star" toward making every decision and with every program and service you provide.

The GEE Method philosophy establishes exactly how we are going to approach each situation with clients and the ACM System is the foundation to the most effective way of influencing the behaviors and changes necessary for our clients to achieve extraordinary results. I will be the first to tell you that the complexity of human movement is something I will always be in wonder of and continuously pursue deeper understanding of. It would be naïve for me to believe I know everything about injury prevention, recovery and human performance. I have my own mentors that bring insights and newer perspectives to light for me as well.

To truly grow and be the most effective at your passion for helping others, it is essential that your mindset be geared toward continuous growth and learning. The GEE Method and ACM System provides a platform to establish the philosophy for what you truly are working toward with your patients and clients. With a defined philosophy and proven approach like ACM, you can begin to remodel your current practice and become part of the necessary paradigm shift in the health care and fitness industry.

The Look Good/Feel Good Gap

One of the biggest questions I ask personal trainers is, "How do you differentiate yourself from the rest of the trainers out there?" The fitness professionals who have achieved higher levels of education and understanding are already differentiating themselves. A fitness enthusiast relies on esthetics and portraying the image of a fit and healthy body. I agree that you must walk your talk, but the perspective toward influencing the general public on health and fitness as "looking good" is completely wrong and not working.

There has never been a time more than now that demands the most qualified health care and fitness professional – here's why.

Obesity, chronic pain and opioid drug abuse are at epidemic proportions in America and having a tremendous impact on our society and culture. A few alarming statistics will illustrate that this growing problem is a responsibility we all share.

Overweight Adults and Obesity

Obesity continues to rise at an epidemic rate as reported by the CDC, Center for Disease Control.

- More than 1 in 3 adults were considered to be overweight.

- More than 2 in 3 adults were considered to be overweight or obese.

- More than 1 in 3 adults were considered to be obese.

- About 1 in 13 adults were considered to be extremely obese.

- About 1 in 6 children and adolescents ages 2 to 19 were considered to be obese.

- More than one-third (36.5%) of U.S. adults are obese.

- Obesity-related conditions include heart disease, stroke, type 2 diabetes and certain types of cancer, some of the leading causes of preventable death.

- The estimated annual medical cost of obesity in the U.S. was $147 billion in 2008 U.S. dollars; the medical costs for people who have obesity were $1,429 higher than those of normal weight.

https://www.cdc.gov/obesity/data/adult.html

Chronic Pain

An analysis in 2012 from the National Institutes of Health shows that Americans are in pain and the problem is growing:

- An estimated 23.4 million adults (10.3 percent) experience a lot of pain.

- An estimated 126 million adults (55.7 percent) reported some type of pain in the three months prior to the survey.

- Adults in the two most severe pain groups were likely to have worse health status, use more health care, and suffer from more disability than those with less severe pain.

- Pain affects more Americans than diabetes, heart disease and cancer combined.

https://www.nih.gov/news-events/news-releases/nih-analysis-shows-americans-are-pain

https://nccih.nih.gov/news/press/08112015

https://report.nih.gov/nihfactsheets/ViewFactSheet.aspx?csid=57

Opioid Drug Abuse

The U.S. Department of Health, the CDC and others report in 2016 the alarming data of the growing epidemic of prescription pain abuse and overdose: 1 out of 5 patients are prescribed opioid drugs for non-pain related diagnoses.

- Primary care provider's account for more than half of opioid pain relievers dispensed compared to pain medicine, surgery and physical medicine and rehabilitation specialists.

- The rate of opioid prescriptions nearly quadrupled from 1999 to 2014, but the rate of Americans suffering with chronic pain remained relatively the same.

- 11.5 million Americans misused prescription opioids

- 116 people in the United States die every day from opioid-related drug overdoses (heroin, etc.)

- 45% of people who used heroin were also addicted to prescription opioid pain killers.

https://www.cdc.gov/drugoverdose/data/prescribing.html,

https://www.asam.org/docs/default-source/advocacy/opioid-addiction-disease-facts-figures.pdf

https://www.drugabuse.gov/about-nida/legislative-activities/testimony-to-congress/2016/americas-addiction-to-opi-oids-heroin-prescription-drug-abuse

https://www.hhs.gov/opioids/about-the-epidemic/

https://www.cdc.gov/vitalsigns/heroin/index.html

If the promotion to look good was working, why is obesity continuing to grow at alarming rates? If getting in shape and lifting weights was the answer, then why are so many Americans suffering from chronic pain and becoming dependent on dangerous drugs for relief? These are the questions we all should be asking ourselves. Is what we are promoting in the health care and fitness industry working?

The image to look good is still the central focus in the fitness industry and the majority of promotional campaigns and marketing strategies are focused more on those individuals who are already fit.

This was a topic of discussion 20 years ago in college, and the problem with the promotion of health and fitness is still not working for the general public.

A large majority of individuals are under the misconception that they need to get into better shape. I'm not saying this is not important or incorrect. It's what this message is saying in general. What does getting in better shape really mean? To the unassuming general public, bombarded with body images of health and fitness, this perception is intimidating and seemingly impossible for most to imagine. Again, if you don't believe it's possible or you don't think it's worth it, you will not pursue it.

This problem is propagated by the image of fitness and health being about esthetics and not about how one feels, or toward a direction that someone believes is attainable. Walk into any gym in America and you see fit bodies everywhere. Sure, you will find some individuals there who are embarking on a fitness quest for the first time, but the majority of health club memberships are purchased by those who have already established a health and fitness lifestyle.

I was having a conversation with one of my friends at the gym about how it feels like everyone is watching you as you lift and he said, "It's the gym. You have to expect to be judged just walking through those doors." As a person who values exercise and a healthy lifestyle, even I feel the judgement and perception that I am being evaluated by my physique at the gym. This is something you just grow accustomed to as part of the scene. To the average person who is simply trying to get in shape, this stigma is overwhelming and discouraging.

The corporate fitness trend has never really taken hold in America. The benefits of getting employees engaged in fitness programs demonstrates improved productivity, reduced absenteeism and overall employee morale; however, less than 10% of employees take advantage of these programs. This reflection of the workforce parallels the reasons most Americans are not engaged in the pursuits of health and fitness, and something needs to change.

There has never been a time that demands the most qualified health care and fitness professional than now. It is our responsibility to be part of the solution with establishing a different paradigm and approach for helping others truly achieve extraordinary results. It must start with determining how to help others believe it is possible, and providing the services and programs that encourage a person to see the value in the efforts you are asking of them.

Filling the Look Good/Feel Good Gap

Two Birds With One Stone

As health care providers and fitness professionals, we understand the many positive side-effects of improving health and fitness. The benefits of exercise and a healthy lifestyle are more specific to an individual's goals and aspirations than what our perceptions are. Promoting the body image is only one small effect and as I have explained, this has not been a positive influence on the general public.

The promotion of health and fitness must to be directed toward what a person can feel and achieve and not on how slim their waist line is or how big their muscles are. The Gee Method and ACM System embody the benefits of health and fitness through influencing a growth mindset toward believing it's possible, and providing a platform for an individual to feel improvement in how they move and function.

I have worked with many clients who ask me how to get six-pack abs or how they can firm up their bodies. The images these clients are coming to me with are centered on how their bodies look. Most of us have self-esteem concerns with the shape of our bodies and an entirely different subject related to where we seek certainty, a topic I will write about in another book – but for now, let's get back to how I work with my body image clients.

I will always take a client through the ACM assessment, regardless of their motivations and goals. Why? Because every client I work with, from those suffering in chronic pain to those who want to improve sports performance or body image, I know it is my duty to provide the most effective results. Those results can still be improving body image, but once a client performs the ACM Assessment, they now can feel where their body may be restricted and where underlying conditions will hold them back.

My clients know that the ability to touch their toes and balance on one leg for 10 seconds is more important than their body image goals and the six-pack abs. I will always encourage clients to exercise, especially if they are motivated to do so, but I emphasize the importance of correcting dysfunction as the main focus in their fitness quests. Without a strong foundation of function, all the motivation and effort in the world will be wasted. At some point these clients will sustain an injury or develop pain that limits their pursuit and eventually deters them from wanting to exercise at all. Enough failed attempts at exercise, and a person begins to believe that it's not possible, and will start the downward cycle I've mentioned so far.

We know that exercise produces results and offers many benefits, regardless of the type of exercise. As health care providers and fitness professionals, we need to be very specific and aware of the results we are working to achieve with our patients and clients. A focus on helping a person – regardless of their goals – to improve underlying movement pattern dysfunctions and postural compensations, will only build a strong foundation for them to continue striving for greater results in fitness. This is what The GEE Method and ACM System promote. The ACM System is the foundation to any aspect of health and fitness pursuits, and the most effective way to establish sustainability with your clients, both physically and mentally.

As we come to the end of this first section of the book, you will notice that I introduced you to a new perspective toward treating patients and working to improve the health and fitness of your clients. To be the most effective in your professional career, and with the patients and clients you are working with, it is essential that you establish a philosophy for the methods, programs and series you offer. You must be aware of the influence you are having in your industry and with your patients and clients. The GEE Method is a philosophy based on higher standards and principles to guide your decisions and influence the greatest change, both in your profession and with your patients and clients.

You've discovered some of the greatest gaps that prevent you or your patients and clients from achieving extraordinary results, and how The GEE Method and ACM System fill those gaps. I've tried to illustrate the laws of cause and effect as they relate to your current approach and the influence this has on the results you are seeing and influences these methods have on our industries and the general public.

Every decision made with the programs and services you offer must be guided by a strong philosophy and purposeful awareness to make the greatest impact physically and mentally with your patients and clients. The second section of this book discusses in detail how the ACM System offers an approach that embodies The GEE Method principles. The ACM System and corrective exercise programs offer you an entirely new approach toward achieving a greater purpose and establishing a direction that will guarantee you are making the most tremendous influence on your industry and with your patients and clients.

PART 2

ACM
Corrective Exercise Programs*

I can't believe just doing these simple exercises worked! This is one of the most common statements we hear from our clients that work with us at ACM and for those who are introduced to ACM for the first time. What is it about corrective exercise therapy that is so successful and leaves clients amazed at the results they get?

The foundation and core belief at ACM is to engage our clients and give them the knowledge, guidance and resources to help them establish their role and responsibility in their own injury prevention and recovery process. We accomplish this through developing the mindset for growth and possibility, while providing the most sustainable results that are not limited with dependency or restrictions. ACM's corrective approach is founded in exercise. We believe that specific exercise

---

The ACM System should never be used as a medical diagnosis nor should it replace or be a substituted for appropriate medical care. A certified exercise therapy specialist must adhere to the scope of practice of their current profession at all times. The ACM System is designed specifically to help healthcare and fitness professionals identify underlying movement pattern dysfunctions and postural compensations in their clients. If you are working with a client who has a history of or experiences discomfort, pain or injury in specific joints or has related orthopedic conditions it is always advised to check with your clients treating physician before performing the ACM fundamental movement assessment.

progressions, designed for each client's particular needs are the most effective way to accomplish freedom from pain and injury.

We are aware that there are many forms of corrective therapy, and believe that each has a role in a client or patient's progress. We work closely with physical therapists, athletic trainers, chiropractors and fitness professionals who share our values in helping patients and clients succeed. We believe that success is not creating dependency on someone else to get better, or restricted to a device or certain product that must be used indefinitely. We work toward supporting our clients and showing them how to help themselves in their injury prevention and recovery process.

The ACM Corrective Exercise program is one of the most effective approaches at re-establishing faulty movement patterns and postural compensation that lead to pain and injury, while providing the foundation for your client's long-term success. As an ACM Certified Exercise Therapy Specialist, you will have the knowledge to determine your client's most underlying movement pattern dysfunctions and provide a corrective approach that offers the precise exercise sequencing to achieve remarkable results.

There are a few concepts that form the foundation for how results are achieved through exercise, whether that is corrective exercise or any type of exercise or training. Those results can be both biomechanical, a change in posture, position and function, and neurological, the science behind increased strength, coordination and stability. As an expert in corrective exercise therapy, you must understand that biomechanical and neurological changes are not only a result of the exercises and training programs we perform, but in large part due to everything we do with our body on a daily basis.

The S.A.I.D. Principle

The S.A.I.D. Principle is an acronym for Specific Adaptation to Imposed Demand, and states that the human body will adapt to the specific demands placed on it. This is the first concept that we must examine to understand the effects of exercise and the results achieved.

The S.A.I.D. Principle implies that performing the same movement repeatedly, whether it is through exercise or physical demands, will have an adaptive effect on our body for that specific skill or activity. A person who performs in a specific sport must train within the demands of that specific sport or activity to improve. The skill and strength necessary for performing the bench press exercise does not transfer to the skills and athleticism of an NHL hockey player or to any athletic performance, for that matter. This is where the concepts of Functional Training started to take hold in the strength and conditioning profession and fitness industry, which we will discuss later.

The human body is highly adaptable to the environment it functions in. Beyond exercise, it is important to understand that everything we do with our body imposes demand, and over time our body will adapt to the specifics of that demand. I always say that we are creatures of habit. We perform tasks over and over again the same way without realizing we are doing it. These habits create adaptation in postures and movement patterns that we perform or don't perform.

Take, for example, kneeling down to pick something up off the floor or stepping up onto a short stool. Nine out of ten times you will always lead with the same leg. This pattern of movement has become a habit and produces the result of one leg being more stable and stronger and a reason why you continue to use the same leg over and over. You are adapting to what you do all day. As one side gets stronger and more stable, the other side is not adapting equally.

One of the most common and alarming examples of adaptation to our environment is the person who sits all day, your child at school or your client who works behind the computer all day. Sitting postures produce a specific imposed demand that our body begins to adapt to. If you observe a three- or four-year-old child, they do not slouch when sitting – if you are able to ever catch them sitting long enough, right? As that child starts going to school, their body is subjected to sitting for extended periods of time each day. Eventually their posture adapts to the demands and position of sitting. Those strong postural muscles they used for running, jumping and playing are no longer supporting them, and we begin to see that damaging slouched, rounded back and shoulder posture. Later in life, these poor postures and limited movement patterns begin to show up as discomfort, pain and injury.

It is critical as a corrective exercise specialist, health care or fitness professional, that we understand the environment our clients are interacting in, the habits they have adapted to and how these demands play a role in their functional capabilities. The S.A.I.D. principle applies to everything we do with our bodies, not just exercise. As an ACM Corrective Exercise Specialist you are going to begin to recognize habitual patterns with your clients as they walk into meet you, stand and talk with you, et cetera. You will notice that they always stand on one foot, rarely shifting their weight to the other side, or that one shoulder is higher than the other. All of these subtle postural adaptations are compensated patterns that offer you clues to how your clients are going to perform during the ACM Assessment, and what to pay attention to during training programs you have designed for them.

Are you really helping your clients succeed, or are you hurting them without even knowing? One of my favorite things to do at the gym is watch people lift weights and perform all the various exercises with the free weights and exercise equipment. I notice the subtle things, like where their foot placement is while bench pressing. I notice if they are standing with their feet even, or are their feet staggered, and if they switch feet. I look at their overall postures performing bicep curls, back rows or shoulder presses.

Good or bad, you are going to get results. Can you tell the difference? Based on the S.A.I.D. Principles, I know for certain that whatever you are doing for exercise you will get results. When you are finished with the set of whatever exercise you were doing, you either improved your mechanics and posture or reinforced the poor mechanics and posture that ultimately led to discomfort, pain and injury. I call the gym ACM's R&D department.

As I have mentioned and will reiterate, the S.A.I.D. principle states that our body will adapt to the specific demands placed on it. If someone is performing a cable crossover exercise for their chest and their feet are staggered, right foot in front of the left, they are reinforcing their ability to stand with their right foot in front, even though they are only working "chest." When I perform the cable crossover exercise, I will always stop halfway and switch my foot position to ensure I am producing the same demands on both sides of the body, fully understanding that it's not just my chest that is working in that exercise.

The next time you are training your client on a specific upper body exercise pattern, take a look at the position their feet are in. I can guarantee you will notice that their feet are pointed out or even worse, one foot points out more than the other. Most people don't pay attention to these subtle but critical details, because they are working their upper body or something seemingly not related to their foot position. Although you may be working a specific muscle group for the day, we can never take away the imposed demands placed on the entire body during that exercise and the adaptive effects that exercise will have overall.

One of the biggest misconceptions in exercise is the ability to isolate muscle groups. I hear everyone talking about which body part they are working today. It's their chest and arm day, and yesterday was back and shoulder day. I agree that you can work on specific muscle groups, but you can never isolate that muscle group. Your entire body is working to stabilize the work performed at a specific muscle. Try lifting your arm straight in front of you, even without weight. If you pay close attention, you will feel work or tension through your back, abs and even legs. Someone who does shoulder presses or bicep curls, isolating their shoulders or arms, will still be producing work throughout the rest of their body.

So to create the most isolation, someone will rest their hands, back, body and even head – yes I've seen this, on a bench or machine. Now, they believe they are getting the most isolation. A great example is the "preacher curl" bench. You rest your elbows, upper Humerus, on a slanted bench and perform the bicep curls, completely isolating the biceps. Ever watch someone perform preacher curls? What are their feet doing? What posture is their back and shoulder position in?

Weight benches and machines are making you weaker, not stronger. So, what is wrong with isolating specific muscle groups? This is what all that fancy gym equipment and machines are for, right? Targeting specific muscle groups for the most effective workout – it's been a concept in the fitness industry since Jack LaLanne opened his first fitness studio in Oakland, California in 1936. Most people measure the effectiveness of a health club or fitness center by the amount and type of equipment it has. The more pieces of fitness equipment the health club has, the better it must be, right? It makes selling memberships much easier and gives trainers a system or protocol to follow to get through each training program with their clients.

Because of my experience working in physical therapy, one of the corporations I was consulting with asked me to interview physical therapy clinics in their area to determine which clinic would be the best solution for the corporation's injured worker's program. The corporation wanted to know which clinic I felt would best prepare their employees for their return to work status. I went to three or four clinics and examined their facilities, recognized most of the equipment they were using, and had a sense about their overall approach they took in the treatment of patients – but I hadn't been sold.

"This is the one," I said ecstatically to the corporate safety manager I was touring facilities with. She was shocked, and said, "How do you know? We haven't even taken the tour yet." It was the fifth clinic we walked into, and I had only walked through the door and introduced myself to the receptionist. The clinic was a huge open space with no treatment tables or fancy gym equipment and modalities like ultra sound or e-stim machines. I could see from the front desk that this physical therapy clinic was different than the four others we had just visited and knew that this is what got people better.

The clinic didn't have the typical rehab machines. This clinic had weights, kettle bells, various types of resistance bands with racks and apparatus along the walls where patients performed functional exercises. During our tour, fully knowing this was the clinic I was going to recommend, I was reassured that they had the traditional modalities and treatment tables but they were isolated in the back rooms.

Their philosophy was on getting people to move again and that meant through specific and functional types of exercise. To this day, almost ten years later, this clinic continues to be the one that the corporation sends their injured workers to because of the results they produce.

As you exercise, lift weights or perform any type of training, the body must create stability during the work. The example of raising your arm up in front of you illustrated that the spine, abs and legs must coordinate a series of muscle contractions to stabilize and counter balance the movement the arm is creating. If you sit on a bench and perform the same movement, the bench is now acting as the stabilizer, and your strong stabilizing postural muscles no longer are recruited for the help.

Any time you place your body on a bench or stabilize your back against the back rest of a machine while performing an exercise, you are shutting off the core stabilizing muscles, not to mention the strong hip and lower extremity muscle groups. The bench or machine becomes your stability now. The problem is, the bench or machine doesn't follow you home, help you do things around the house or help you perform as an athlete. You are getting weaker as your extremities, those beach muscles, get stronger. The body cannot work effectively like this, and eventually, the weaker posture will no longer support even the simple tasks you want to perform.

Don't misunderstand me. Personally, I like lifting weights. I like lifting heavy weights. However, the difference is that I challenge each of the exercise patterns, or incorporate as much instability into my routines and exercises as possible. I only perform one exercise on a bench, the chest press with dumbbells. If you watch anyone perform this movement, they spread their feet wide, create a big arch in their back and press the dumbbells up and down together. How can you create instability in an exercise that is essentially very stable?

I place both my feet on the bench or up in the air, taking the stability of the floor away, and perform the chest presses one arm at a time, alternating right, then left, each rep. As one arm lowers, the other is holding the weight above my chest. I am creating an added challenge to the pattern and causing my body to stabilize the rotational effects of each arm moving independently. Sounds easy, huh? Every time I do this exercise, I have someone ask me why. They are only looking at the chest involvement and ask me if it's a better isolation. I explain to them the effects of the exercise on the entire body and how it benefits them beyond chest isolation.

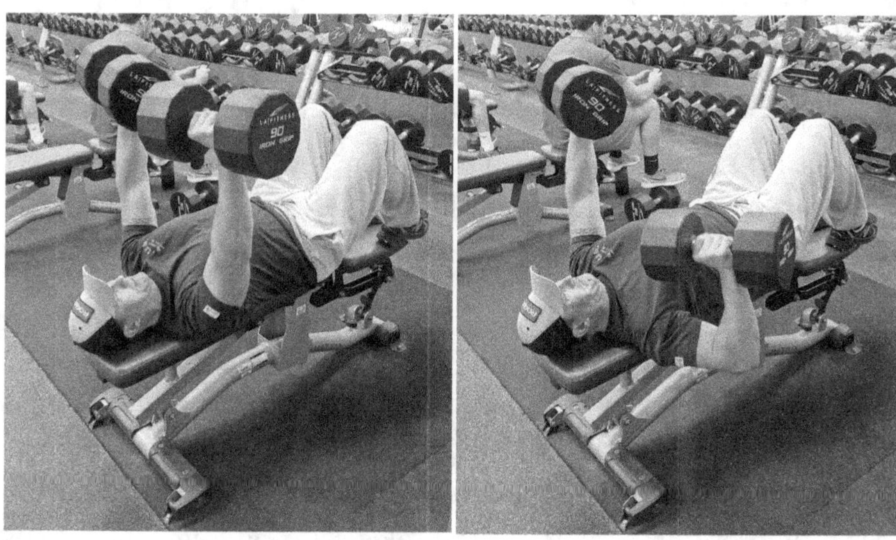

After showing this movement to some of my friends and the guys who ask, I observe them trying it and one of my friends actually fell off the bench. Each one of them says, "That's way too hard." Isn't that the focus of exercise? To work the weakest link? They all revert back to the wide base of support with their feet and making the exercise as easy as possible – and later come to me asking what I can do to help them with their back pain.

As an ACM Corrective Exercise Specialist or health care and fitness professional, it is important to understand the concepts of adaptation. You must recognize how every activity, exercise and task you and your clients perform is having an influence on a positive or negative outcome for physical performance.

The S.A.I.D. principle applies directly to corrective exercise therapy because you are focusing on the specific movement pattern dysfunction and postural compensation to be corrected. The ACM Fundamental Movement Pattern Assessment will help guide your corrective exercise approach by giving you a clearer understanding of the dysfunctions that have caused the limited adaptations your clients are presenting. The ACM Corrective Exercise Programs promote the specific movement pattern adaptations through the demands of specialized exercise sequences. You will have the knowledge and certainty as an ACM Certified Exercise Therapy Specialist that the corrective approach is achieving the positive results that your clients will notice and value.

The Overload Principle

The Overload Principle is the second concept we need to discuss as it relates to the results of exercise and how those results apply to the benefits of corrective exercise specifically. The Overload Principle states that to improve physical and/or neurological conditioning, the body must be exposed to a greater stress or demand than it is accustomed to. Progression is the key to the effectiveness of the Overload Principle and is what the ACM Corrective Exercise approach establishes. As an ACM Certified Exercise Therapy Specialist, you will have the knowledge to accurately assess your client's greatest dysfunctions and provide the most relevant specific demand and progression to their corrective approach.

"Work is work," said one of my college professors, who was helping settle a debate between a few of my friends and me. We were studying exercise physiology and trying to determine the most effective amount of sets, reps and types of exercise to produce the biggest gains in muscle growth according to science. I still remember that one comment he made. All three of us sat there with a blank stare on our faces; it was our introduction to the overload principles of exercise.

"It doesn't matter what you do," he said, "as long as it's more than your body is used to doing." That statement ended our debate immediately and became the foundation for how we looked at exercise and fitness all together. We no longer looked at the machines and equipment in the gym the same again. It was this concept that really solidified my understanding of corrective exercise and how to be the most effective at producing sustainable results.

As an athletic trainer working in the college systems with Division I athletes, I was always amazed at some of the athletes' freakish size and strength, only to be humbled by the nagging injuries many sustained to areas of the body so minimal compared to their apparent athletic abilities. The strength and conditioning coaches understood the Overload Principle and pushed these athletes hard. It appeared that everything was working great! Apply more work to the athlete than their body was capable of, and they achieved improvements in strength, endurance and power. However, what we as athletic trainers saw were the injuries, and some were so perplexing to me.

I remember one athlete, a football running back whose arms and shoulders were bigger than my head. This guy was a monster and played like it, too, but he came to me one day very concerned about the shoulder pain he was experiencing. It was then that I realized although the Overload Principle was in full effect with this guy's training, there was a missing component that was never addressed.

You are only as strong as your weakest link. This Division I football player, who ended up making it to the NFL for many years, had rotator cuff damage. His shoulders were massive, strong and solid, but the weaker supporting rotator cuff muscles were completely overpowered and getting weaker. This is where the overload principle in corrective exercise applies. You must impose demand to the weakest link first before building the bigger and stronger structures. Performing shoulder presses does not ensure you are working the weaker and deeper structural muscles like the rotator cuff. It's why, if you've ever had a rotator cuff injury or know anyone who has, they are given these simple band exercises to perform, specific to rotator cuff function, not the deltoid strength and size.

Training the weakest link is what truly makes you stronger. As my career expanded into the corrective exercise field, I began to understand even more how important it was to identify the weakest links and establish a solid foundation to build from. I had employed the Overload Principle and progression through every workout I performed at the gym and in my athletic conditioning. The problem was, I continued to get injured, and my athletic performance never seemed to improve.

I knew that I needed to take a step back, and for an athlete that was not easy. Initially, I was in the same place most of our clients begin. How are these simple exercises going to help me? I needed to trust my knowledge of anatomy and biomechanics. I needed to trust the extensive research and personal experiences I had throughout my athletic and professional career. I was certain that I had discovered something that nobody else had. You've read my story and the journey I was on to solve the knee problems that plagued me my entire life. Once I stepped back and trusted the corrective exercise process, I was never more confident. The progression from limitation and pain to improved athletic performance and injury recovery gave me the assurance to push myself harder with my training. Every day, I check my weakest links and evaluate where I am physically, to ensure I am working on what needs to be done first.

DJ is a client of ACM and came to us with a genuine concern. He works in law enforcement with the government and appears visually strong and imposing. Putting it mildly, DJ has some impressive muscle growth and strength. He mentioned that he was dead lifting over 500 lbs., and his squat was close to that. His concern was the pain he was experiencing in his left hip, knee and ankle and seemed to be getting worse. His workouts had dropped off and he didn't know what to do.

We performed the ACM Fundamental Movement Pattern Assessment on DJ and uncovered a few distinct limitations specific to his ankles and hips. After seeing the results of the ACM Assessment, DJ was convinced that this was the problem. He was confident in moving forward with the prescribed corrective exercise program we had developed for him. Six (6) exercises are all we gave him to do.

Compared to the workouts this guy was doing, he was not impressed with these simple corrective exercises, although he trusted what the ACM Assessment told him. We suggested laying off the weight room for a while until he had worked on his corrective approach. This again was not easy for him to commit to, but he did.

Each week, DJ checked in with us on his progress, and he was slowly seeing improvement in the limited movement patterns, and the pain was subsiding in his ankle and hip. We prescribed his progression to the initial corrective exercise program, and he worked on that for the next week or two with more excitement that something was happening.

A month into the program, it was time for DJ to face his fears about going back into the weight room. As part of his progression, he needed to test the patterns that the ACM system was re-establishing. Below is the actual email we received from DJ after five weeks of working with the ACM Corrective Exercise Programs we had prescribed.

> *"I haven't forgotten about you, just been doing the exercises and was kind of scared to get back under the bar for fear that the program wasn't working, even though the hip pain has definitely subsided.*
>
> *Today I did front and back squats (back squats worked up to 285 for 8) and didn't feel too much of any pain (last rep or so I felt some tenderness). The best depth I've gotten in both in a long while and the best I've felt in them as well!"*

It's not a matter of if; it's a matter of when. As you begin working with your clients, you must be aware of their postural compensations and movement pattern dysfunctions before you begin placing demand on their structures with your training program. This is why the ACM System is critical for anyone in the health care or fitness industry. Your clients are coming to you with poor postures and movement pattern limitation that they have adapted to and been reinforcing their entire lives. If you are not correcting these limited movement patterns or postural compensation first, you are only going to reinforce them further and cause more damage.

Corrective Exercise

The concept of Corrective Exercise is nothing more than understanding the S.A.I.D. and Overload principles and applying then to the body in a way that reinforces or produces positive results in mechanics, posture and function. Everything we do with our clients is going to produce a result, period. It is your responsibility to understand if that result is a positive experience for your client, or if you are hindering performance and creating compensated postures and faulty mechanics that will ultimately lead your client to pain and injury.

Corrective Exercise works! It follows the guiding principles of adaptation and overload progression to achieve positive results, if you have identified the underlying movement pattern limitation and postural compensations accurately. The ACM assessment system, along with our exclusive corrective exercise programs deliver the most effective approach toward identifying those weakest links and a proven approach toward achieving sustainable and extraordinary results.

The adaptation and progression principles make it clear that the effect of corrective exercise is proven results. One of the most challenging aspects to corrective exercise is understanding where to begin. We have a corrective exercise library of over 460 exercises and growing every day. How do you determine which exercises are going to have the greatest effect and produce the most sustainable results?

One of Michael Gerber's most important concepts in his book, *The E-Myth Revisited,* is, "If you do not have a system for your business, you do not have a business." He explains that to be successful in business, you must have an operating procedure or system that runs the business. The ACM System is exactly that – an operating procedure to identify the most underlying movement pattern dysfunctions and determine the most effective corrective approach for your clients. The ACM System takes the guess work and wasted time out of performing a movement pattern assessment and helps you to determine the most effective corrective exercise approach.

It has taken over 20 years of study in anatomy, biomechanics and injury prevention and recovery to begin to have a strong understanding of the complexity of human movement and function. ACM provides a system that can be replicated from one exercise therapist to another and from one client to another. The ACM System takes away much of the intuitive aspects to corrective exercise therapy that other methods insist is the only way to learn. The ACM Fundamental Movement Pattern Assessment can be measured and objectively compared to previous assessments to determine the effectiveness of the corrective exercise approach.

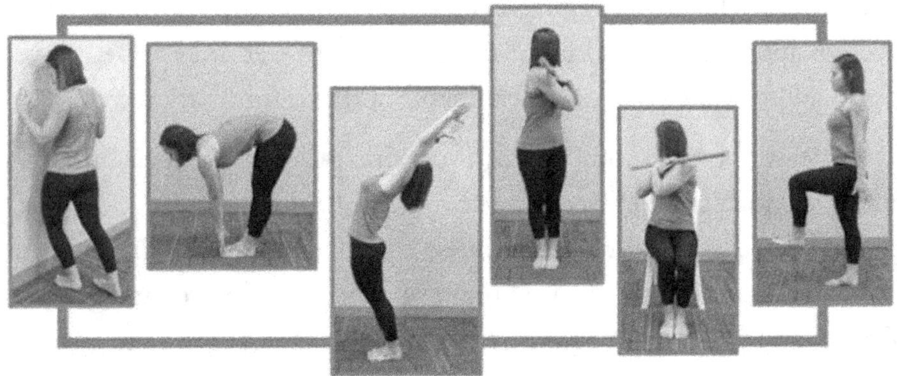

What is the ACM Corrective Exercise Program system and how does it work? The ACM System begins with the assessment. Our Fundamental Movement Pattern Assessment is the initial phase of the system of corrective exercise. We must first understand what we are trying to correct before we can understand the most effective approach. Our ACM Certified Exercise Therapy Specialist course details each fundamental movement pattern assessments and how they play a role in determining the most underlying dysfunctions.

I have studied many of the postural correction methods and movement pattern screens in my career. I was never confident in the approach because as I have mentioned, much of it was left up to intuition, and having years of experience that could not be replicated from one therapist or client to the other. Each therapist had their own interpretation for the postural compensation they identified. Given the same client, another therapist would have an entirely different perspective toward the corrective approach.

I knew that there had to be a more objective way of determining a client's postural compensation and an approach that could be replicated. Working with hundreds of thousands of clients over the past 20 years, I began to recognize patterns and realized that postural compensation or what most of us refer to as poor posture, was a result, not the cause of a deeper problem. Poor posture and postural compensation is the end result of what we do or don't do well each day and that is move.

The chicken or the egg, which came first? Some would argue that postural compensation causes limited movement patterns, and there is some accuracy in that assumption after the fact. If we continue to dig deeper into the question which came first, keeping in mind the design of the human body and the developmental phases of upright posture and movement, we get a clearer understanding of which came first.

We are designed for movement first, with joints that are highly flexible and without restriction. Through the early years of development, we learn to stabilize that movement efficiently and effectively. Our attempts at standing upright on two feet require the coordination of over 640 muscles that control roughly 200 bones. Everything must work in unison and harmony to move throughout our environment. At an early age the design is correct, there are no limitations to movement, and given the correct stimulus or specific adaptive demands, such as crawling and upright walking, our body develops the natural postures that support and move us.

To gain an even greater appreciation for these developmental stages and the consequences of skipping a stage you must read ***Original Strength***, by Tim Anderson and Geoff Neupert.

Poor posture is a result of an inability to move correctly. Think back when you were a baby first learning to crawl, or observe a baby who is just starting this stage of development. You do not have to teach them to crawl, they figure out the most effective and efficient way possible. As they begin to own this movement pattern, as Grey Cook would say in his book, ***Movement,*** they have now earned the right to stand.

This is where things go terribly wrong. Eager parents begin to encourage their child to stand on two feet and attempt walking long before they are structurally ready. The body must make the necessary neurological connections to the 640 muscles of the body and coordinate those muscles at the precise time to establish the necessary balance between mobility and stability in an upright posture. When we skip this step in development, our babies still stand and learn to walk as we all did, but they find another way. We recruit different motor programs and use muscles that are not specifically responsible for the task they are being asked to do. This is where some of the movement pattern dysfunctions and postural compensations begin.

We place babies in all kinds of apparatus that help them walk on two feet. These apparatus are equated to the gym equipment that we discussed earlier in this chapter. The devices help stabilize the body and provide a false sense of strength, stability and security. Over time, our body will adapt, but will find another way to adjust for the lack of correctly-acquired strength and stability necessary for even the most basic movement patterns. As a result of applying external support to stabilize inefficient posture, either as babies to help us walk sooner or in the gym and rehab setting to isolate or build strength to specific muscles, our body will continue to work, but finds another way. The body must find a way to move even if it is inefficient or dysfunctional. Our body will always find the path of least resistance, but at a sacrifice. We can only perform this way for so long before something gives out.

Arthritis, tendonitis, torn ligaments, degenerative disc disease, and the list of chronic pain disorders goes on. These terrible conditions that plague our lives, in most cases, can be related back to a dysfunctional movement pattern that became a postural compensation. The assessment of postural compensation is only the surface of what is happening below and to determine the most underlying condition associated to a person's poor posture we must examine the ability or inability to move correctly.

The ACM Fundamental Movement Pattern focuses on the most basic patterns of movement that are the foundation to higher level functioning movements. It's always interesting when one of our clients asks us why they can still perform high level movements with some of the dysfunctions we determined in our ACM assessment. All we do is remind them why they came to us in the first place. In most cases it's because they have either seen a decrease in their athletic performance or have some type of injury or nagging chronic pain condition. We tell them it's possible to perform higher level exercises, but only for so long before something gives out. If you do not own the most basic movement patterns first, you are finding another way to perform that violates the body's design and results in breakdown, compensation and eventually pain and injury. Remember our discussion on training the weakest link?

We've discussed how performing very select exercise sequences can have a tremendous effect on correcting movement pattern dysfunctions and postural compensations. You have learned that the human body will adapt to any stimulus, as long as that stimulus is specific, greater than what the body is accustomed to and follows a progressive change. This next section will focus on exactly how we select and determine the most appropriate corrective exercise sequences and programs.

Start with the Purpose in Mind

BUY, BUY, BUY!

Have you ever watched the financial news, specifically Mad Money with Jim Cramer? He is that highly energetic guy who is always hitting his "BUY, BUY, BUY" or "SELL, SELL, SELL" button when callers ask him for specific stock advice. Before you get worried, I'm not about to start giving you investment advice, except to say investing in yourself will always have the greatest payoffs! The reason I bring up Jim Cramer is because of the commercial that advertises his show, Mad Money. Google "Mad Money Commercial" and watch.

Jim walks down the street and observes people eating lunch and riding their bike. As everyone is saying "Booyah" to Jim, he begins to analyze what they are wearing or the types of consumer goods they are using. It's like the Terminator scanning the person, and Jim sees these people very differently. He equates the Nike shoes as a stock price and the Prada purse as a buy or sell limit. His expertise of investment banking and financial advice has him seeing the world differently.

As you continue to develop the knowledge and understanding of movement pattern dysfunction and postural compensation with the ACM System, you will begin to identify the most subtle problems in your patients and clients. You are going to analyze your patients and clients just like Jim Cramer analyzes stock prices of individuals walking down the street. With every movement, exercise and position your patients and clients perform, you will begin to see subtle compensations and dysfunctions that otherwise you would have never noticed.

The true power of ACM is developing the awareness and knowledge to identify dysfunction and postural compensation in everything your patients and clients are doing.

I have a client who was explaining to me about his recent knee pain following a run. He explained that his wife runs, and he wanted to start running with her. Following the most recent run, his knee really started to hurt. As he explained his story to me, he sat down to show me where it hurt and pinpoint the exact spot. It was his left knee that was hurting, but I noticed as he sat in the chair, his right leg was in a completely different position than his left.

A chair provides a balanced and symmetrical foundation for our hips placement, right? The chair was nothing fancy and very little seat cushion, so I knew it wasn't the chair that was influencing this asymmetrical posture. His right foot was twisted out to the side almost pointing at a 45-degree angle from his right knee. Sounds painful, huh? He wasn't even aware of it, and when I asked him to turn his right foot inward, pointing in the direction of his right knee, even with the left, he said it felt strange and not normal.

I told him to go back to the way he was sitting, get comfortable. Immediately his right foot twisted outward compared to his right knee. Then I told him to forget about his feet and knees and to just sit up straight arching his low back. Without looking at his feet his right foot "miraculously" turned in the direction that his knee was pointing. I told him to look down and he was shocked. It didn't feel uncomfortable now.

What did all of this observation tell me? It told me that his left knee pain, which I quickly steered his attention away from, was coming from a greater problem. I mentioned that he should ice the inflamed knee and give it a rest, but my focus was on explaining that his right hip was not functioning like the left, at least while he sat in a chair. I asked him if he only runs left footed and after a laugh, he said no. I explained that if his right leg and foot are doing something different while he sits, wouldn't the same conclusion be logical when he ran, a much higher level of demand? He immediately asked me what he could do about his right hip! His focus was off the left knee pain, and he quickly understood that his right hip function was really the problem with his left knee.

Performing the ACM Fundamental Movement assessment with him revealed what that one observation told me. We were able to narrow down to where this subtle dysfunction was coming from and had a clear direction for an effective corrective approach. Where do you think most would have started in treating his left knee pain? Most likely stretching the muscles of the left hip and knee – because after all, that's where his pain was, right?

The ACM System is your baseline assessment to detect even the most subtle dysfunctions or postural compensations and gives you the insight on where to start your corrective approach. The deeper your awareness is and the greater your knowledge becomes in identifying movement pattern dysfunctions and observing postural compensation, the more effective you will become at truly helping your patients and clients achieve extraordinary results.

The ACM Corrective Exercise System

We have developed a step-by-step process for determining the most relevant corrective exercise approach for the dysfunctions we have identified with the ACM Fundamental Movement Pattern Assessment. This protocol is based on the understanding of anatomy, biomechanics and injury prevention and recovery research. Following the ACM protocol will help you make more informed decisions on where to focus your attention and offer better guidance in working with your clients.

It can be challenging to stay focused on the correction of the movement pattern limitations and postural compensations that you have identified with the ACM Assessment protocol when your clients have specific areas of discomfort and concerns. We have worked with thousands of clients who have areas of pain that make it challenging for them to understand why we work on their ankle mobility or non-specific body parts as the overall corrective approach.

There are times you will want to focus on something obvious, like a person who has a forward head position and rounded shoulder. Both types of postures are very easy to identify and draw our attention away from the purpose of the corrective approach, especially if that person is experiencing discomfort or pain in the shoulders or neck. As an ACM Certified Exercise Therapy Specialist, you will understand that their symptoms are only a result of a deeper problem. When you have identified obvious postural compensations, you will have the knowledge to educate your clients on the overall corrective process and immediately generate results they can feel and see.

The ACM corrective exercise protocol follows a progressive model for establishing mobility symmetry, then stability symmetry. We follow that natural developmental model for human movement that was instinctual from the time we were born. We had all the mobility we ever needed and lacked any way to control or stabilize that movement. Over time, three or four years, we established the stability or control while maintaining all the great mobility we were born with. During those early years, we challenged the simple patterns of movement and progressed to higher-level movement patterns like running and jumping. One of my favorite sayings to clients when asked about their progression is, "You must crawl before you walk, and you must walk before you run." That simple statement is the foundation to the ACM corrective exercise protocol.

We establish where the greatest mobility restrictions are in clients and understand that a lack of mobility around a joint limits the function or control of that joint. You can't strengthen a joint and ensure its optimal function if it can't move effectively. This is why we always want to understand and identify any mobility restrictions first.

You will discover while performing the ACM Fundamental Movement Pattern Assessment with your clients that many people have mobility restrictions. They will even tell you that their hamstrings are tight or their calves are tight. They may tell you that they stretch all the time, or they know they need to stretch, but don't. This is one of the greatest myths and misconceptions related to identifying tight muscle groups.

For example, you may have heard of the condition called "sciatica." The term refers to nerve (the sciatic nerve) pain and numbness that begins in the gluteal area and runs down the back of the leg to the knee. If you Google or search YouTube for the term "sciatica" you will most likely come across what many call "Piriformis Syndrome." Piriformis Syndrome is simply a condition where the piriformis muscle, one of the deep six external rotators of the hips, becomes excessively tight. The piriformis muscle is blamed for the sciatica pain because the sciatic nerve runs very close to or in some cases through the piriformis muscle.

During your search you will come across half a dozen "piriformis stretches". The majority of the healthcare and fitness professionals understand that tightness of the piriformis can contribute to sciatica and that stretching this muscle alleviates the symptoms. Sounds good on the surface; who doesn't want to be out of pain, right? As an ACM Certified Exercise Therapy Specialist you will learn that we do not focus on tight muscles – rather, we focus on WHY that muscle got tight. A tight muscle just means it's been working harder than it's supposed to. Sure, there could have been an injury, surgery or some type of condition that causes that specific muscle to shorten; however, that is not the case most of the time. It is important to understand that a tight muscle, whether it is the piriformis or hamstrings, is only tight because something else is weak.

If you only stretch a tight muscle, you haven't addressed WHY it's tight, only relieved it temporarily. The ACM Corrective Exercise programs do not focus on stretching tight muscles. We focus on understanding what muscles may be ineffective at performing their job, forcing other muscles to overcompensate and perform a job they were not intended to perform. This concept is one of the most important lessons to learn as an ACM Corrective Exercise Therapist. Depending on your level of education, training and experience, this concept may be very hard to abandon. I am a perfect example of that. It took me years to finally give into the fact that stretching my tight hamstrings was not the most effective way to achieve touching my toes. Once I started to focus on weaker stability muscles and dysfunctional movement patterns, my hamstrings miraculously released.

Once you have established a greater range of motion through a joint, the key is to maintain and challenge that range of motion. Teach the body what to do with that new movement. If you are fixed on stretching a tight muscle, fine, I am not going to stop you. However, you better teach the body what to do with that new movement or it will go right back to what it already knows, the motor program it has already established around a limited joint.

Stretching tight muscles may feel good after and you may have better range of motion for a short period of time. This is what makes the ACM Corrective Exercise Program so valuable. Once we re-establish movement, our exercise sequences are designed to reinforce that movement and teach the body what do to with it afterwards. This means the tight muscles can go back to doing their job while the surrounding muscles are activated to get to work again.

Knowing how to establish the improved movement pattern, then reinforce and train the body how to use it effectively is what makes the ACM Corrective Exercise sequencing so valuable. We are able to establish authentic movement that is reproducible through the specific exercise progression in each corrective program.

The ACM Progressive System Approach

At ACM, our approach towards corrective exercise is based on three very specific progressive phases. These phases for an individual's progression are specific to their physical conditions, goals and level of commitment. Each phase of the ACM corrective exercise program is designed for progression from one phase to the other. The corrective approach varies depending on where our clients fall into one of the three categories of function.

The most beneficial features of the ACM Fundamental Movement Pattern Assessment System are to identify the movement pattern limitation and postural compensations before they start to contribute to pain and injury. Our primary goal with ACM is to help prevent pain and injury; however, many of your clients are already experiencing pain or have sustained injuries that limit their physical abilities before you have the opportunity to work with them.

When a person suffers from pain or injury they usually get a prescription from the doctor. At ACM, we believe the corrective exercise program is their pain pill to address the true causes of pain related to movement pattern dysfunctions and postural compensations. This provides our clients with a resource that is beneficial, non-addictive and sustainable.

Category I: PRO-Scriptive Phase

Clients who have been experiencing chronic pain or sustained an acute injury or state a subjective pain levels above a five (5) out of ten (10) are considered to be in our first category, the PRO-Scriptive Phase. In this category, we still try to perform the entire ACM Fundamental Movement Pattern Assessment and note which, if any, of the movement patterns cause pain and where. You have to understand that if your client is experiencing pain, an authentic movement pattern cannot be expected. Pain can cause an excitatory or inhibitory muscular response, and all bets are off when assessing authentic movement patterns.

We may be able to determine from just a few movement patterns that do not cause pain if there are dysfunctions or limitations that could be a contributing factor. Our ACM Exercise Therapy Certification course prepares you to understand each movement pattern in detail and how each is closely associated with the next. You may have a client experiencing low back or neck pain and performing the Ankle Mobility Pattern and Standing Rotation Pattern does not cause pain but leads you to understand more about where someone may have deeper dysfunctions.

Many times, with our clients in pain, we start at a lower-level progression exercise. Simply laying a client on their back and having them perform some of our supine exercises will relieve their symptoms. Remember, the goal as an ACM Exercise Therapy Specialist, even with symptomatic clients, is not to diagnose or treat the pain. We are using the corrective exercises to have an influence on their posture and movement pattern limitations. Pain does not limit our scope of exercise selection, their postural compensations and movement pattern limitations are what direct us. We have had clients with severe acute disc herniation's find relief in a wall sit exercise. As an ACM Certified Exercise Therapy Specialist you will have the knowledge and understanding to know when an exercise is appropriate and when it is not. Simply by watching a client perform the exercise, you will notice subtle compensations or limitations that are influencing a negative response with the exercise.

As your client progresses with their corrective exercise program, their symptoms will diminish. You must continue to perform the ACM Fundamental Movement Pattern Assessment on your client continuously as their symptoms diminish. Each time you perform the assessment, you are getting a deeper understanding of their capabilities and they are gaining the necessary confidence to move pain free again. When our clients have reached a pain-free level or have a subjective pain level less than four out of ten, we begin to progress their corrective exercise program. This could happen in one session or ten sessions, but as you recall, the success of exercise is based on progression and this is the most important aspect to corrective exercise therapy.

Category II: PRO-Daptive Phase

As clients progress from the PRO-Scriptive Phase, or when we work with clients who are not experiencing pain, it is critical to assess their movement capabilities. We call this category the PRO-Daptive phase. As you may guess, we named this phase after the S.A.I.D. principle, Specific Adaptation for Imposed Demand. The adaptive phase, or as we call it the PRO-Daptive phase, is our chance to identify where postural habits and limited movement patterns have caused dysfunctions and compensation on clients who are not limited with pain yet. I like to say, "The signs of pain and injury are already there, long before the actual symptoms show up."

The focus of the PRO-Daptive phase of corrective exercise is centered on providing the specific exercise sequences and a level of demand that will create positive changes in the movement pattern dysfunctions you have identified. During the PRO-Daptive phase, it is important to continuously re-assess your clients after each exercise or program. We do not want to assume the exercises are going to work. With the ACM Fundamental Movement Pattern Assessment, you can obtain objective results immediately. If an exercise or sequence was not effective at improving the dysfunctions you were working on, do not waste your client's time. Find the right progression, sequence and demand that imposes the greatest adaptation. Many times those changes may be subtle; however, it's progress in the right direction.

You will find that the majority of your clients will fall into the PRO-Daptive Phase of corrective exercise therapy. Do not be overconfident that because your client is not experiencing pain or they have progressed from the PRO-Scriptive phase that they aren't at risk. Remember, we named this category PRO-Daptive because whatever you do in this phase, the result will be an adaptation in one direction or the other. You must ensure your clients are adapting in the right direction. Paying close attention to their efforts during the exercise programs is critical. If you see subtle compensations or shifts in their body as they perform the exercise program you have selected, you are not re-establishing a good pattern, you are reinforcing the poor pattern they already have. This means the progression and demand level of the exercise program is more than they are able to handle. Take a step back and establish the correct pattern, even if that means reducing the demand and load.

I spend some time at the gym working out, as I have mentioned. Many members will ask me questions about an exercise they saw me performing because it was a little different than what they were taught to do. A gentleman that I befriended while working out one day was on the leg press machine. He has become a good friend, and I was joking with him about how much weight he had on the machine. He had over 900 lbs. loaded on the sled, and I told him to leave some weights for the rest of us to use. After a laugh, he started to ask me questions about why I never do the leg press machine. In my opinion the leg press machine is one of the most useless and damaging exercises one can perform at the gym. I generally leave my opinions to myself, but when people ask me why I'm doing a particular exercise, I will tell them.

He was intrigued with my explanation about the leg press, and asked me if I could perform the ACM Assessment on him. He had no pain, and he is a pretty avid weight lifter. He is extremely muscular, and as I mentioned, can push a lot of weight on the leg press. When I took him through the ACM assessment – that only took about 3 minutes – he had impressive mobility for a large muscular man. When I took him through the stability sequence, simply standing on one foot for ten seconds, he couldn't balance to save his life. I gave him three attempts on both feet and you should have seen him. He looked like a tight rope walker in a wind storm without the large stability pole they carry.

That portion of the assessment shocked him, especially when I said, "So, is the leg press helping or hurting you?" The explanation about the leg press I shared with him started to make a lot of sense. I told him that even though he can press over 900 lbs. he couldn't even stand on one leg. If the leg press was such a great strength building exercise, why wasn't it helping his stability? Because the leg press provides the stability with a large back rest and places the hips and legs in a position that does not simulate any type of functional movements. Stunned, he asked me how he could improve the stability problem he has. I told him he needs to earn the right to load the body. Reluctantly he asked, "So I probably shouldn't be doing the leg press?" I didn't have to explain anymore to him. He understood the progressive phases of corrective exercise.

It's important to understand that we cannot expect perfection. Most of us all have varying levels of mobility or stability dysfunctions with postural compensations. It's extremely valuable and important to understand where yours or your client's are to keep a keen eye out for adaptation in the wrong direction. I have worked in corrective exercise for over 25 years, and as you recall, it all started with trying to fix myself. I have a few movement pattern limitations, very few, but they are there. I work on my corrective exercises daily and without them I wouldn't be walking today, let alone running marathons and performing the higher level activities that I do. Even if you have established functional scores in the ACM Fundamental Movement Pattern Assessment, it is always important to re-assess often to ensure your body is moving in the right direction, pun intended.

Category III: PRO-Formance Phase

The last category in our progressive phases of corrective exercise is called the PRO-Formance phase. This is the highest threshold level of corrective exercise, movement and performance. At this level we are imposing even greater demand, challenging the good patterns of movement we have established. The human body is amazing at adaptation. We know in medical research that following an injury to an elite athlete, their muscular endurance and strength diminished by more than half in the first month of immobilization. The majority of your clients may not be elite athletes and you may only see them a few times a week for workouts or therapy. What are they doing the rest of the time? Remember when we discussed understanding the environment your clients is exposed to. Are they sitting all day at work, then in their car and then when they get home? Can you expect the adaptive changes you established during your session with them to stick if they are not challenging those greater patterns of movement? The answer is certainly no.

This is why it is still important to perform the ACM Fundamental Movement Pattern assessment throughout your client's progression through the phases of corrective exercise. The PRO-Formance phase is where functional training programs have the most benefit for clients. Just performing functional exercise doesn't make you functional. Remember you are going to either restore or reinforce a movement pattern. At the higher level thresholds of exercise, your body must be able to perform without thinking. The correct pattern should be established before you try to load it.

I am asked all the time by clients and friends at the gym how to perform a deadlift exercise correctly. They watch me performing a deficit deadlift. That means I am standing on a four-inch platform and going deeper than normal. It intrigues people and they want to know how and why. I simply pull them away from the weight rack and ask them to touch their toes. More than half the people I work with like this have extreme limitation is the hip hinge pattern of touching their toes. Their backs round excessively with little movement from the pelvis. I show them in the mirror and demonstrate what a hip hinge toe touch should look like. I simply say you shouldn't deadlift until you can touch your toes.

During a deadlift, too many things are happening at once. It is impossible to attempt a heavy deadlift and be thinking about moving correctly. If you are able to reproduce a good movement pattern unloaded, then I say progress to a loaded pattern like the deadlift. If you continue to deadlift with an inability to touch your toes, you are only going to reinforce the faulty motor program and eventually injure yourself or your clients.

The PRO-Formance phase of corrective exercise is about challenging movement patterns from simple to complex and being aware of any dysfunctions or compensation that arise. Take a step back, reinforce a good pattern then challenge it. It's something I do daily. Between my runs and my workouts, I am highly aware of what my body is doing, right or wrong. When I run, I cannot pay attention to how my foot is hitting the ground, my knee alignment and my torso stabilization for very long. Running patterns are highly complex and happen in a split second. So how do I know if I've established a good patterns or reinforced bad patterns? I know the next day. Some of my runs are long and hilly. I get sore, and I pay close attention to where I am sore. Is the soreness bi-lateral or do I have pain in only one calf or quad? I look at my running shoes often to determine if my heel strike and toe off are the same on both sides of the sole or is one different. All of these observations lead me to understand if my running pattern is good or bad. If something is off, I don't wait; I begin correcting the pattern at a lower level then go test it in a run again.

Taking a client from the PRO-Daptive phase to the PRO-Formance phase of corrective exercise is highly dependent on your client's goals and how quickly their body can re-establish an authentic movement pattern. One of my biggest assessments I perform every morning and throughout the day or during workouts is the toe touching pattern. Once I was able to establish my toe touching pattern, I knew it was going to be very important for me to continue to reinforce the movement pattern. If there is anything I'm doing in my workouts or in my environment that limits or reduces my ability to touch my toes, I correct it immediately. As you may recall, the inability to touch my toes is what led me to nearly having my knees replaced at the age of 27. It is highly important for me to maintain that pattern and re-assess through my day.

To summarize the categories of corrective exercise, the PRO-Scriptive phase is intended for those who are suffering in pain and have sustained an acute injury with a pain level greater than five out of ten. The PRO-Daptive phase is intended for those who are not experiencing pain or who have a low level of pain that does not interfere with authentic movement patterns. This phase is where you will be strongly re-establishing movement pattern limitation you have identified. The PRO-Formance phase is simply the progression into higher level threshold exercises that challenge the authentic movement patterns. You will find people that gravitate between the two latter phases, like I do. I challenge higher-level patterns, but always go back to the PRO-Daptive Phase of corrective exercise to ensure I am moving authentically at the lower-level demands.

The ACM Corrective Exercise programs are designed to have the greatest influence on those clients who are relatively pain free and fall into the PRO-Daptive or PRO-Formance phase of corrective exercise therapy. We apply the same principles, techniques and systems to our clients who are in pain or have sustained an injury. In our PRO-Scriptive phase, however, the exercise sequences and level of demand meets the client's functional capabilities, which at the time may be very low. Remember that our focus is not on fixing symptoms but on fixing the underlying conditions that cause the pain and injuries people suffer from. We provide the same components of our corrective exercise protocol to our clients who are suffering in pain or injury, with the same principles as we apply to those in the more advanced phases, only at a different level of demand.

How to determine corrective exercises

One of the most frustrating tasks that I had to perform while working in physical therapy was picking out of a deck of index cards, the home exercise program for my patients. Each pack of index cards was sectioned off for which body part you were working on and the intended purpose of the exercises; for instance, range of motion or stability. We then had to place each card on a copy machine and print the page. If you were to look at anyone's home program they received from their physical therapist, chiropractor and massage therapist for example, you would most likely be able to guess what the person's problem was, or at least where they had pain.

When you look at an ACM Corrective Exercise program you will not be thinking about where a person's pain or symptoms are, but what the outcome or purpose of doing this specific sequence of exercises is to accomplish. You may see an ACM corrective program for someone who has neck pain and the focus on their specific program is on ankle mobility.

Say what?

Looking at the entire kinetic chain from the law of cause and effect is a skill you will begin to develop as you embrace the purpose for everything you do from a movement pattern and postural compensation problem. Whether you are using a deck of index cards, exercise photos from a website provider or what you have stored in your mind from the years of experience of working in your field, it is critical that the focus on your exercise selection and the sequence of exercises you provide are aimed at progressively improving the most underlying movement pattern dysfunctions and postural compensations.

At ACM, we utilize over 460 different corrective exercises that promote adaptation, progression and sustainable change in movement patterns and postural conditioning. From the 460-plus different corrective exercises in our library, we determine the most relevant exercises that will have the greatest influence on our client's current physical limitations and condition.

Determining which exercises from the 460 different exercises we utilize can be overwhelming if you do not have a plan to initiate the corrective approach with your clients. The ACM System helps you determine where to start in the correction of movement pattern dysfunctions and postural compensations you have identified, with an objective and measurable result to test your program against.

It is important to understand that any exercise can be a corrective exercise if utilized effectively. Our exclusive corrective exercise library continues to grow with variations of exercises and progressions that we test and find useful in the corrective approach. The key to determining which exercise to choose is in understanding how that exercise influences the movement patterns or postural change you are working on.

One of the most important aspects to our ACM Corrective Exercise programs is in the sequencing or order that we put each exercise in. Just like our system to determine which movement pattern dysfunction to begin correcting, we must have a system for determining which exercises to choose and which order they are in for the corrective exercise program. The protocol for determining which movement pattern dysfunction we focus on first is based on understanding the influence each specific movement pattern limitation has on pain, injury and postural compensations.

The corrective exercise selection protocol we have developed is based on the principles of exercise adaptation and progressive demand, previously discussed, along with the general knowledge of anatomy, biomechanics, exercise physiology and postural compensation. Our ACM Exercise Therapy Specialist Certification course provides the knowledge and background necessary to become effective at corrective exercise selection.

Here is an example of a corrective exercise program sequence:

- Static Back Pullovers

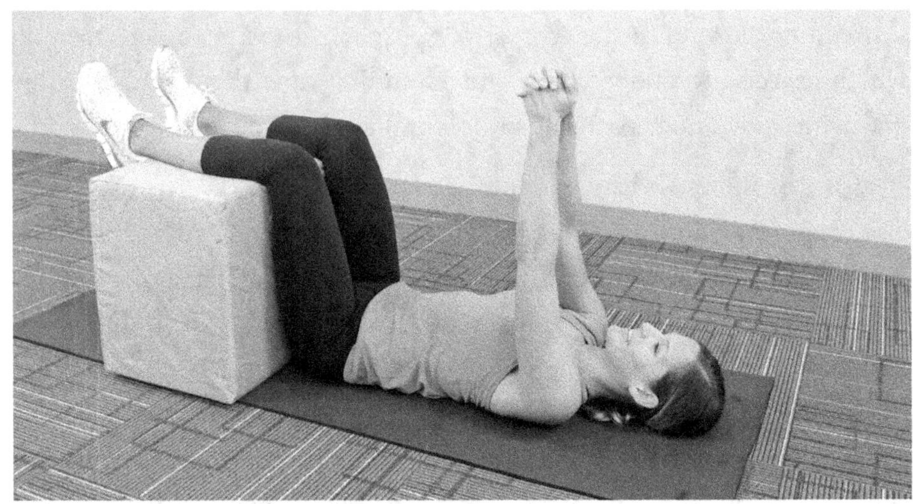

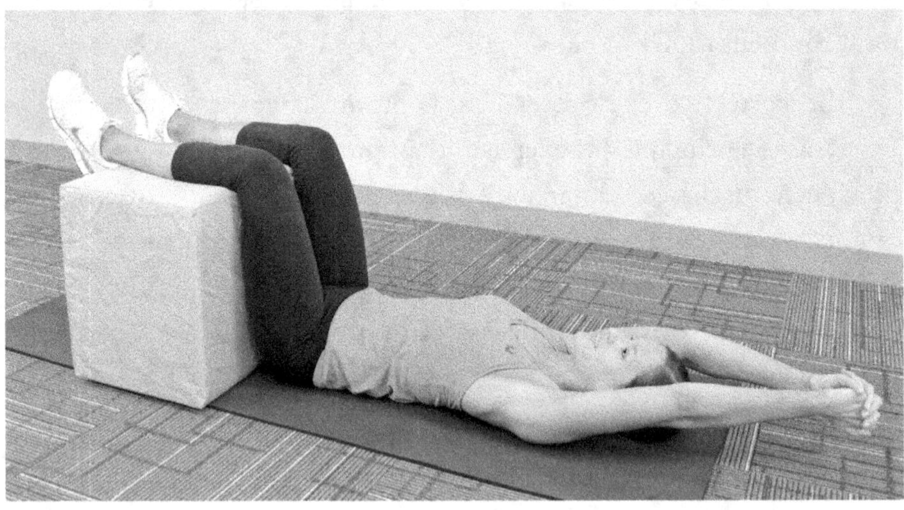

- Supine Foot Circle - Point Flexes

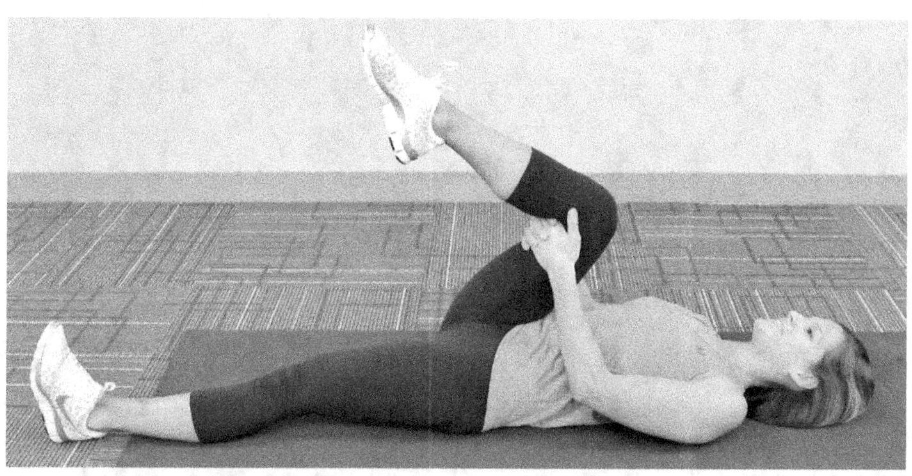

- Active Frogs

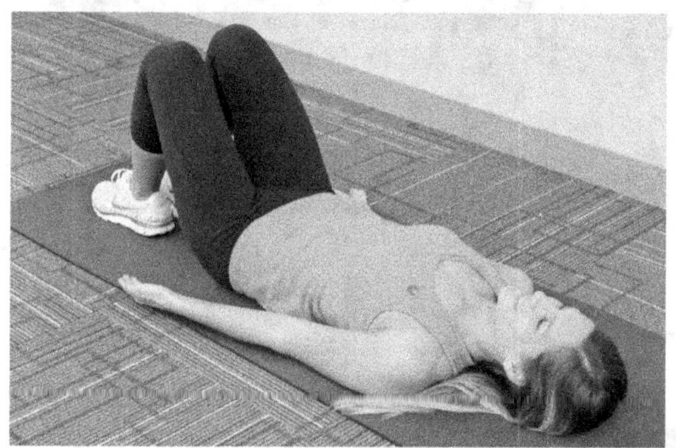

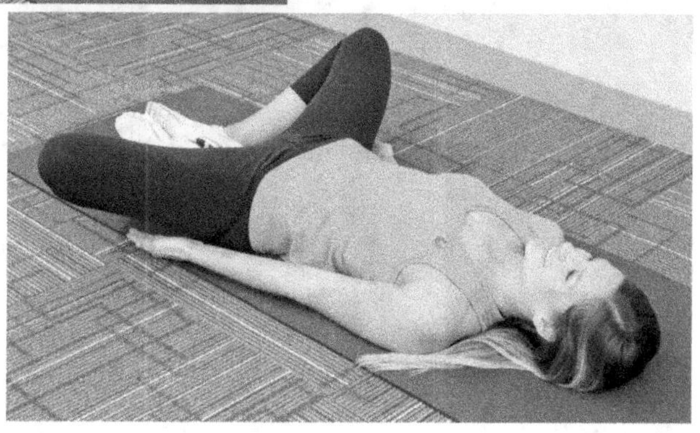

- Supine Active Straight Leg Raises – Presses

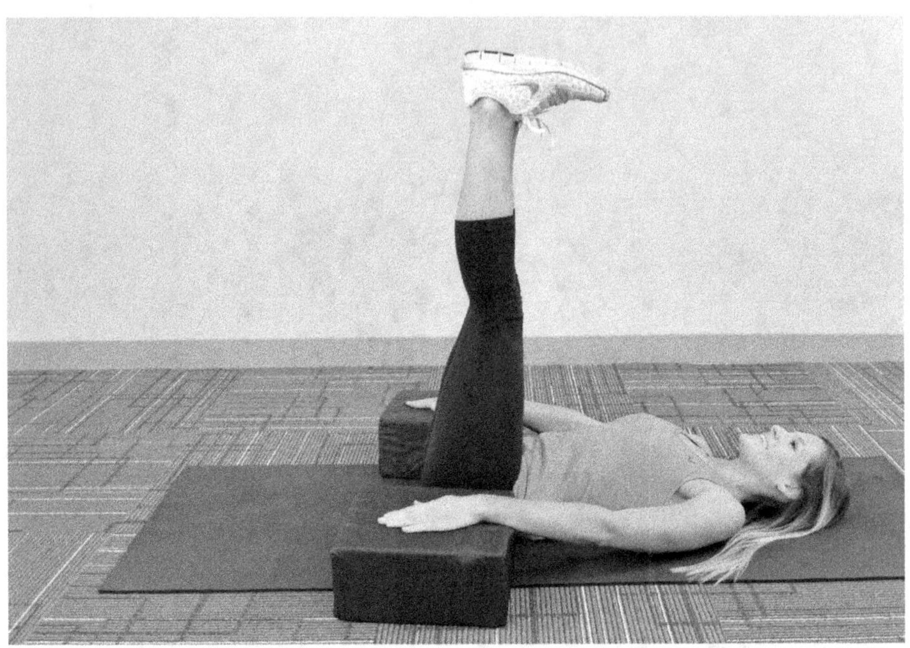

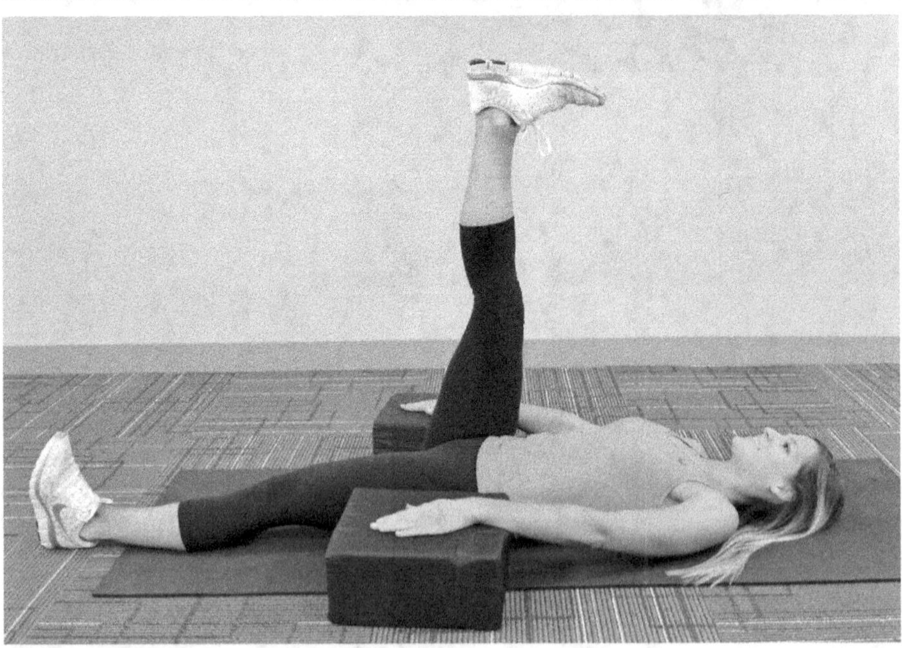

- Hip Hinge – Wide Stance

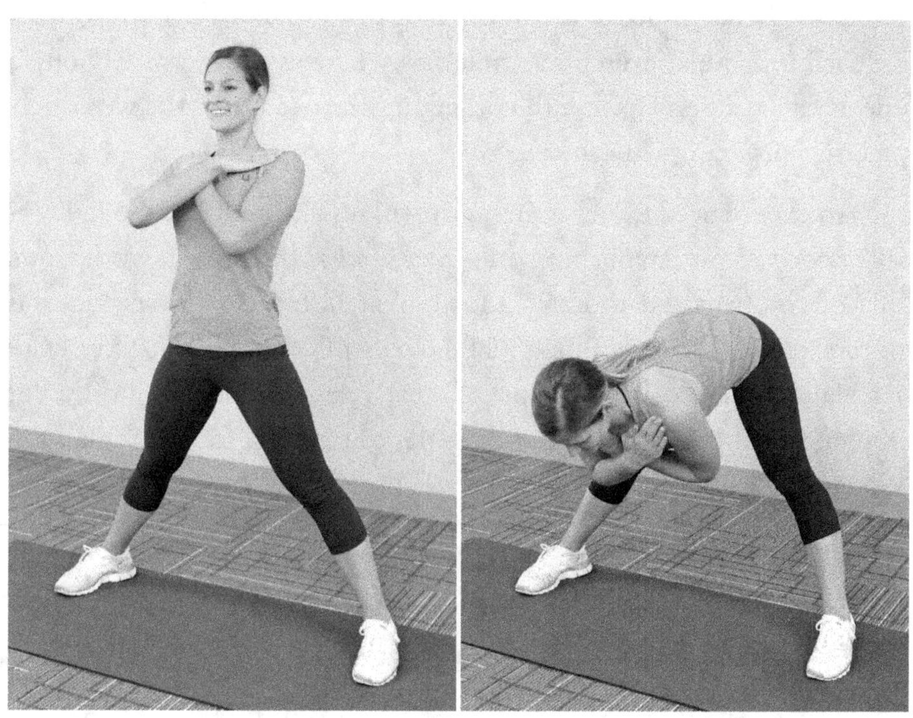

- Kneeling Ankle Squeeze – Presses

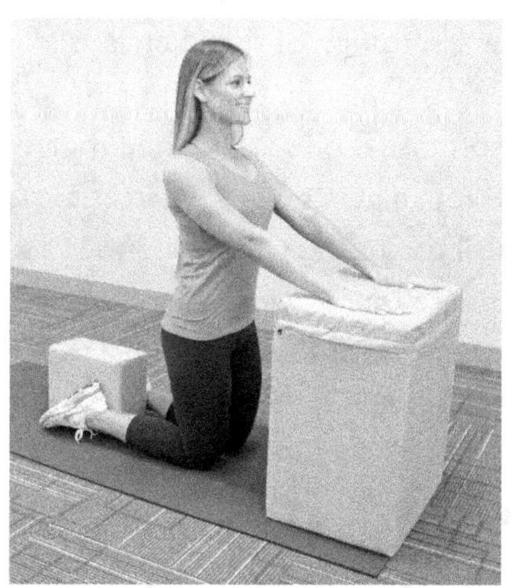

To most people this looks like a list of exercises, to an experienced Exercise Therapy Specialist it reads like a paragraph. We do not focus on each individual exercise as much as we focus on the collaborative effects each exercise has on the other and the overall results we anticipate this program will achieve.

An experienced exercise therapist will understand that the first exercise focuses on establishing a foundation for the hips to work from, free of compensated thoracic and lumbar influence. The second and third exercises focus on functional movements of the hip sockets from a bi-lateral and unilateral approach, each exercise having a different influence, but collectively providing the foundation for the remaining exercises.

The fourth exercise in our corrective exercise sequence example begins to add demand to the hips where we have facilitated better movement. The last two exercises help us establish how the body is to use or interpret the new movement. It's like locking in the new pattern by teaching the body that the movement is correct and should work through the range of motion we are providing.

Nowhere in the description of this exercise sequence did I mention where the injury or pain may be located or that the program should alleviate those symptoms. The focus of the program and focus of corrective exercise therapy in general is to correct movement pattern dysfunctions that contribute to the pain or injuries a person suffers from. An experienced exercise therapy specialist must understand which exercises are contraindicated for the symptoms, pain or injuries a person may have; however, it should influence in the direction of fixing a client's pain.

The first thing an ACM Exercise Therapy Specialist must learn is how to perform each exercise correctly. As they learn each exercise, they must pay attention to every aspect of that exercise, and not just the obvious. If I asked you to perform a bicep curl in the gym, and then asked what muscles were working, most people would say the biceps, the obvious purpose of a bicep curl. As an ACM Exercise Therapy Specialist, you will have the insights to understand that the biceps are working, sure, but also the muscles of the shoulder girdle, erector spinae and even lower extremity, to name only a few.

The ability to look at exercise, any exercise, from a different perspective will give you the greatest advantage at understanding corrective exercise progression and sequencing. As we have discussed, isolating muscles is a common misconception, because the entire musculoskeletal system is inter-reliant on each individual muscle and joint as a whole. As you gain a deeper understanding of exercise, you must be looking for the muscles that are working and also the muscles that are not working, that should be, as part of the entire system.

A great example of this is your standard shoulder exercise, the military press. The majority of people perform this exercise sitting with their back supported on the back rest as they press the barbell or dumbbells overhead. The noticeable observation would be that the shoulders are being isolated, which in some case is true. However, to raise your arm overhead, as you do in the military press, the muscles of your spine, abdominals and hips must be activated to stabilize the lumbar spine. Pressing your back against the back rest weakens these strong postural muscles and predisposes you to injuries of the spine and shoulder.

I perform a variation of the shoulder press, although I get into a half-kneeling position with one knee on the ground and the other foot in front of me. I place the forward foot as close to my midline as possible without falling over. Using the opposite arm as the leg that is forward, right foot forward, left arm lifting, I press one dumbbell overhead. As I work through the motion, my entire body is reacting to the instability of being in an unbalanced and unsupported position. My shoulder is working, yes, and my entire body is working to support the load overhead, unilaterally which challenges the pattern even more. I will also perform a bi-lateral shoulder press with dumbbells following the half-kneeling presses; however, I sit on a bench with no back support. The amount of weight I can lift is limited to the strength of my back, abs and hips. I still get an amazing shoulder workout with the added demand of working my weakest links.

This concept of understanding every aspect and influence an exercise has on working muscles, stretching muscles, deactivated muscles and joint position will transform how you train yourself and your clients. Always consider the weakest link in the entire kinetic chain and work from there forward. At ACM, we never perform a stretching exercise. Although some of our exercises are called "stretching," we are using that exercise for many reasons – to stretch a tight muscle and to also activate weaker muscles that are being facilitated by the position in which the exercise is being performed.

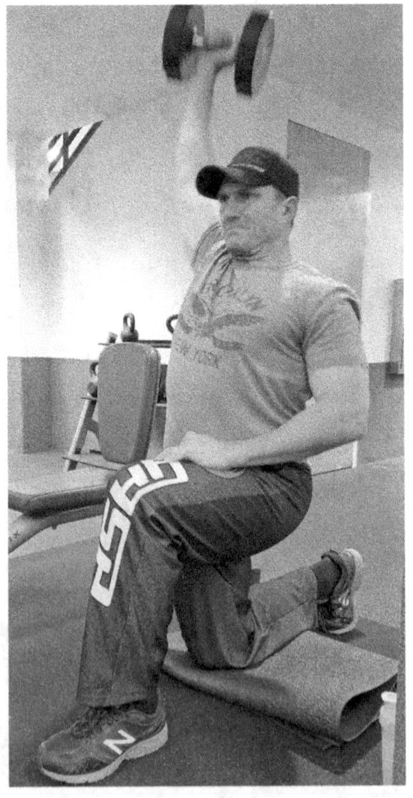

We perform an exercise called the "counter stretch." In this exercise, you will have a client place their hands on a wall or counter at about shoulder height and walk back bending over so their torso is extended and hips over the feet. This exercise appears to be a stretching exercise for their hamstrings. If you asked a client where they feel the work, they will emphasize the extreme stretch of the hamstring; however, we ask them to tighten their thighs and actively arch their back. We are getting muscle activation out of the groups of muscles that oppose the hamstring tightness and placing the spine in a more advantageous position for strength and support.

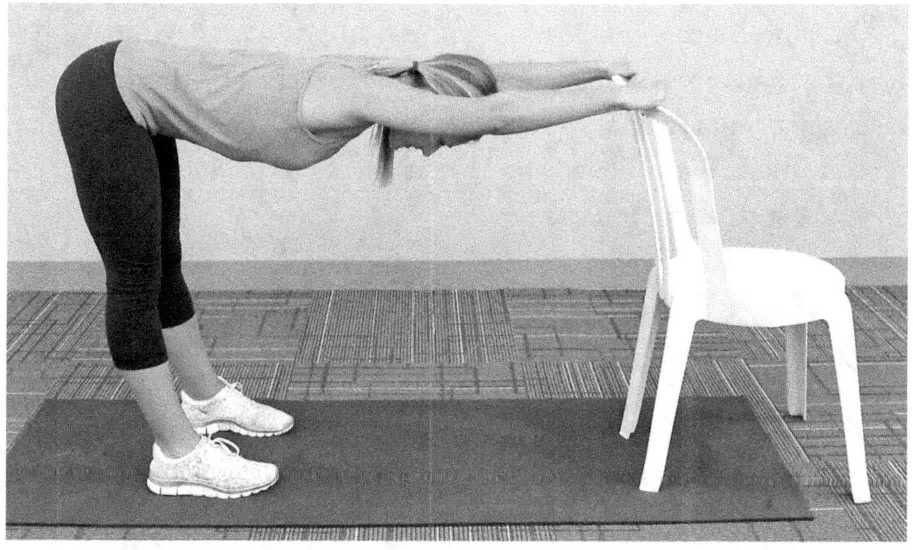

A focus on understanding the influence an exercise has on the entire body is what makes the ACM corrective exercise programs so beneficial and provides the foundation for effective movement pattern and postural change. For every obvious purpose an exercise has, we consider all of the not-so-obvious influences, including muscle activation, deactivation, stretch and joint position. In building a corrective exercise sequence, each exercise may have many different purposes, and combined in the right orders, you will see the body transform with movement patterns and postural compensation improve tremendously.

Our ACM Certified Exercise Therapy Specialist certification course provides the knowledge and background for performing the most effective movement pattern assessment and prepares you to begin learning how our pre-designed corrective exercise programs work with each pattern. As our ACM Certified Exercise Therapy Specialists begin working with clients and providing the pre-designed corrective programs, they are learning how each individual exercise influences change, along with the entire program sequence.

As a health care provider and fitness professional, begin to recognize that every exercise or movement you are having your patients and clients perform is having an influence on the entire body. Many times, when working with clients who have tremendous pain, I will say there is always something you can do.

So, What Now?

The main focus of this book was in connecting both professions of the health spectrum with a central theme and focus. From those who treat illness, pain and injury, to those who work toward improved human performance, we are all connected through the marvelous design of the human body. My experiences as a therapist, trainer and patient gave me the insights for developing a philosophy and system that will be a tremendous benefit to you.

"It's in the moments of decision that your destiny is shaped."

– Tony Robbins

There are times in our lives that require us to make important decisions. Following the conclusion of this book, I believe you understand now that you need to make a decision. This decision involves not only your well-being, but the lives of the patients and clients who put their trust in you. You need to make a decision that is bigger than yourself. Make the decision to become a change leader in your industry with ACM.

Start your new journey with us today by going to www.ACM-360PRO.com/certifications. The accredited ACM Certified Exercise Therapy Specialist course is available there for you online. When you start the ACM Certification course, all of your course material will be readily available in our easy-to-navigate membership site. There are many more features, content and resources at www.ACM360PRO.com, so be sure to get on the site and become part of this incredible program.

If you would like to contact me, please email me at Mike@ACM-360PRO.com. I invite your communication, discussions and inquiries.

"For every sale you miss because you're too enthusiastic, you will miss a hundred because you're not enthusiastic enough."

– Zig Ziglar

One of the biggest reasons most people don't experience the life they truly dream of is because of fear. It isn't easy writing a book and putting your thoughts and ideas out there in the world. My fear wasn't in being judged, my greatest fear was that I had discovered something so important, something that will have such a tremendous benefit to the world, and nobody was going to know about it. This is what drove me to write this book. This is what drove me to invest all of my savings in the development of the ACM System, and this is what drives me to inspire you into taking action.

I encourage you to join me and get involved on my social media sites at www.MikeGee360.com and take advantage of the opportunity ACM is offering you at www.ACM360PRO.com.

I can guarantee that when you embrace the philosophy of The GEE Method and begin to utilize the principles of the ACM System, it will become one of the most transformational and rewarding endeavors you experience as you progress on your journey in your profession and your life.

Thank you for reading.

"In the end, we only regret the chances we didn't take, relationships we were afraid to have and the decisions we waited too long to make."

–LEWIS CARROLL

Acknowledgements

The greatest contributors of this book, who I am tremendously grateful for, and want to say thank you to, are the thousands of clients I've worked with over the years. It was your initial trust in me and the dedication and commitment to yourself that made this book possible and will help many more transform their lives.

I am extremely fortunate for the mentors in my life who saw something different in me and continuously encouraged me to push my own limits of what I thought was possible. You helped me develop the courage to stand up for what I believe in, and the confidence to take on the many challenges along the way.

Those who are closest to me have seen the dedication, commitment and sacrifices I've made toward the pursuits of my dreams and goals. It is your unconditional support, love and the acceptance of the path I've chosen in my life that has given me the strength to continue.

My father, mother and twin sister have been there through it all. Words can't describe the love I have and the sense of gratitude I owe them for being my biggest fans and supporters. Thank you for always believing in me and giving me so much of yourselves to allow me to pursue my life's passion.

The greatest acknowledgement I'd like to make is toward all those who I haven't met yet. Those of you who may be suffering in pain or afraid after an injury, those who don't see the light at the end of the tunnel and are confused with which direction to turn. I can guarantee that the insights and methods in this book will be that light to help pull you through some of those darkest times and provide you a resource of professionals who embrace the principles and philosophy written about in this book.

I am proud to be associated with an industry that strives for continuous learning, innovation and the acceptance that we will always be in awe of the human body's design and function.

References

<u>Books and Articles</u>

Aarass, A., R.H. Westgaard, E. Stranden, Postural angles as an indicator of postural load and muscular injury in occupational work situations. Ergonomics 31 (1988) 6 915 – 933.

Adams, Sieg. (1992) Illustrated Essentials of Musculoskeletal Anatomy (Adams). Megabooks Inc. Gainesville, FL.

Anderson, B. (1997) Stretching at your computer or desk. Bolinas, CA. Shelter Publications Inc.

Anderson T., Neupert G. (2013). Original Strength, Regaining the body you were meant to have. Xulonpress.com.

Araújo F, Lucas R, Alegrete N, Azevedo A, Barros H, Individual and contextual characteristics as determinants of sagittal standing posture: a population-based study of adults, *The Spine Journal* (2014), doi: 10.1016/j. spinee.2014.01.040.

Baechle, Thomas. ESSENTIAL OF STRENGTH TRAINING AND CONDITIONING National Strength and Conditioning Association. Champaign: Human Kinetics, 1994. Print.

Bahrmann A, Zieschang T, Neumann T, Hein G, Oster P. Carpal tunnel syndrome in diabetes mellitus. Med Klin (Munich). 2010 Mar;105(3):150-4.

Berg, K. (2011) Prescriptive Stretching. Champaign, IL. Human Kinetics.

Bigos, Stanley J., MD, John Holland, MD, MPH, Carole Holland, PhD, John S. Webster, MD, MBA, Michele Battie, PhD, Judith A. Malmgren, PhD., High-quality controlled trials on preventing episodes of back problems: systematic literature review in working-age adults. The Spine Journal 9 (2009) 147–168.

Black, Nancy, Leon DesRoches, Isabelle Arsenault, Observed postural variations across computer workers during a day of sedentary computer work. *Proceedings of the Human Factors and Ergonomics Society Annual Meeting* 2012 56: 1119.

Cailliet, Rene. LOW BACK PAIN SYNDROME. 5th. Philadelphia: F.A. Davis Company, 1995. Print.

Callaghan, Jack P., Nadine M. Dunk Examination of the flexion relaxation phenomenon in erectorspinae muscles during short duration slumped sitting. Clinical Biomechanics 17 (2002) 353–360.

Caneiro, Joao Paulo, Peter O'Sullivan, Angus Burnett, Avi Barach, David O'Neil, Orjan Tveit, Karolina Olafsdottir, The influence of different sitting postures on head/neck posture and muscle activity. Manual Therapy 15 (2010) 54–60.

Cheadle, A, G Franklin, C Wolfhagen, J Savarino, P Y Liu, C Salley, and M Weaver. Factors influencing the duration of work-related disability: a population-based study of Washington State workers' compensation. American Journal of Public Health February 1994: Vol. 84, No. 2, pp. 190-196. doi: 10.2105/AJPH.84.2.190.

Chen, Han-Ming *, Chun-Tong Leung, The effect on forearm and shoulder muscle activity in using different slanted computer mice. Clinical Biomechanics 22 (2007) 518–523.

References

Claus, Andrew P., Julie A. Hides, PhD, G. Lorimer Moseley, PhD, Paul W. Hodges, PhD., Different Ways to Balance the Spine Subtle Changes in Sagittal Spinal Curves Affect Regional Muscle Activity. SPINE Volume 34, Number 6, pp E208–E214.

Claus, Andrew P., Julie A. Hides, G. Lorimer Moseley, Paul W. Hodges, 2009 Is 'ideal' sitting posture real?: Measurement of spinal curves in four sitting postures. Manual Therapy 14, (2009) 404–408.

Cook, G. (2003). Athletic Body in Balance. Champaign, IL. Human Kinetics.

Cook, G (2010). MOVEMENT Functional Movement Systems, Santa Cruz, CA. On Target Publications.

Coyle, Edward F., Wade H. Martin III, David R. Sinacore, Michael J. Joyner, James M. Hagberg, John 0. Holloszy, Time course of loss of adaptations after stopping prolonged intense endurance training. Applied Physiology Section, Department of Medicine, Washington University School of Medicine, St. Louis, Missouri 63110; and Exercise Physiology Laboratory, Department of Physical and Health Education, University of Texas, Austin, Texas 78712.

Cristofolini, Luca, PhD, Nicola Brandolini, MS, Valentina Danesi, MEnga, Mateusz M. Juszczyk, PhD, Paolo Erani, BEnga, Marco Viceconti, PhD. Strain distribution in the lumbar vertebrae under different loading configurations. The Spine Journal 13 (2013) 1281-1292.

DeRango, Kelly, Benjamin C. Amick, Michelle Robertson, and Ted Rooney, et al. "The Productivity Consequences of Two Ergonomic Interventions." (2009) Upjohn Institute Working Paper No. 03-95. Kalamazoo, MI: W.E. Upjohn Institute for Employment Research. http://research.upjohn.org/up_workingpapers/95.

Dunk, Nadine M., Jack P. Callaghan, Gender-based differences in postural responses to seated exposures, Clinical Biomechanics 20, (2005) 1101–1110.

Edmonston, Stephen J., Hon Yan Chan, Gorman Chi Wing Ngai, M. Linda R. Warren, Jonathan M. Williams, Susan Glennon, Kevin Netto, Postural neck pain: An investigation of habitual sitting posture, perception of 'good' posture and cervicothoracic kinaesthesia. Manual Therapy 12 (2007) 363–371.

Egoscue, Pete, and Roger Gittines. The Egoscue Method of Health Through Motion, A Revolutionary Program That Lets You Rediscover the Body's Power to Protect and Rejuvenate Itself. 1st. New York: Harper Collins Publishing, 1992. Print.

Egoscue, Pete, and Roger Gittines. PAIN FREE AT YOUR PC. 1st. New York: Bantam Books, 1999. Print.

Falk Mörl, Ingo Bradl, Lumbar posture and muscular activity while sitting during office work. Journal of Electromyography and Kinesiology 23 (2013) 362–368.

Falla, Deborah, Shaun O'Leary, Amy Fagan, Gwendolen Jull, Recruitment of the deep cervical flexor muscles during a postural-correction exercise performed in sitting. Manual Therapy 12 (2007) 139–143.

Fenety, Anne and Joan M Walker Short-Term Effects of Workstation Exercises on Musculoskeletal Discomfort and Postural Changes in Seated Video Display Unit Workers. *PHYS THER*. 2002; 82:578-589.

Flash Anatomy (2004) Joints and Ligaments, Bryan Edwards, A Publishing Company, Inc.

Flash Anatomy (2004) The Muscles of the Head and Neck, Vol 1, Bryan Edwards, A Publishing Company, Inc.

Flash Anatomy (2004) The Muscles of the Head and Neck, Vol II, Bryan Edwards, A Publishing Company, Inc.

Flash Anatomy (2004) The Muscular System, Vol I, Bryan Edwards, A Publishing Company, Inc.

172

Flash Anatomy (2004) The Muscular System, Vol II, Bryan Edwards, A Publishing Company, Inc.

Flash Anatomy (2004) The Skeletal System, Vol I, Bryan Edwards, A Publishing Company, Inc.

Flash Anatomy (2004) The Skeletal System, Vol II, Bryan Edwards, A Publishing Company, Inc.

Fortanasce, V., Gutkind, D. Watkins, R. (2012) End Back & Neck Pain. Champaign, IL. Human Kinetics.

Galen, C. (1998). The chair, rethinking culture, body, and design. New York: W.W. Norton & Company.

Garrick, James, and David Webb. SPORTS INJURIES: Diagnosis and Management. 1st. Philadelphia: Saunders Company, 1990. Print.

Haller, Michael, Christoph Richter, Peter Brandl, Sabine Gross1, Gerold Schossleitner, Andreas Schrempf, Hideaki Nii, Maki Sugimoto, Masahiko Inami, Finding the right way for interrupting people improving their sitting posture. Media Interaction Lab, Upper Austria University of Applied Sciences, Austria Medical Technology, Upper Austria University of Applied Sciences, Austria, Keio-NUS Cute Center, Singapore/Japan.

Hamill, Joseph, and Kathleen Knutzen. Biomechanical Basis of Human Movement. Media: Williams & Wilkins, 1995. Print.

Hamill, Joseph, and Kathleen M. Knutzen. *Biomechanical Basis of Human Movement*, 3rd Ed., USA: Lippincott Williams & Wilkins, 2009.

Hansen, George R., MD, Jon Streltzer, MD., The Psychology of Pain. Emerg Med Clin N Am 23 (2005) 339–348.

Heinrich, J, B M Blatter, P M Bongers, A comparison of methods for the assessment of postural load and duration of computer use. Occup Environ Med 2004;61:1027–1031. doi: 10.1136/oem.2004.013219.

Hetzler B., Rakowski, K., Raynor, J. (2015) MOVEMENT RESTORATION Improving Movement Always And In All Ways. Lexington, KY. Movement Restoration LLC.

Hoppenfeld, Stanley. PHYSICAL EXAMINATION OF THE SPINE AND EXTREMITIES. Norwalk: Appleton & Lange, Print.

Howell, John N., Gary Chleboun, Robert Conatser, Muscle Stiffness, Strength loss, Swelling and Soreness Following Exercise-Induced Injury in Humans. *Journal of Physiology* (1993), 464, pp. 183-196.

Human Factors and Ergonomics Society. (2007). ANSI/HFES 100-2007, human factors engineering of computer workstations. (2007 ed.). Santa Monica: Human Factors and Ergonomic Society.

Jakobson, Cathryn Ramin. (2017) Crooked. Harper Collins.

Jensen, Gail M, Biomechanics of the Lumbar Intervertebral Disk: A Review. *PHYS THER.* 1980; 60:765-773.

Johnson, J. (2012) Postural Assessment. Champaign, IL. Human Kinetics.

Jorgensen, Michael J., PhD, William S. Marras, PhD, Purnendu Gupta, MD, Thomas R. Waters, PhD., Effect of torso flexion on the lumbar torso extensormuscle sagittal plane moment arms. The Spine Journal 3 (2003) 363–369.

Jull G, Trott P, Potter H, *et al.* A randomized controlled trial of exercise and manipulative therapy for cervicogenic headache. *Spine* 2002:27:1835–45.

Keller, Tony S., PhD, Christopher J. Colloca, Deed E. Harrison, Donald D. Harrison, PhD, Tadeusz J. Janik, PhD., Influence of spine morphology on intervertebral disc loads and stresses in asymptomatic adults: implications for the ideal spine. The Spine Journal 5 (2005) 297–309.

Kendall, Florence, Elizabeth McCreary, and Patricia Provance. MUSCLE TESTING AND FUNCTION with POSTURE AND PAIN. 4th. Philadelphia: Lippincott Williams & Wilkins, 1993. Print.

REFERENCES

Kiani J, Goharifar H, Moghimbeigi A, Azizkhani H. Prevalence and risk factors of five most common upper extremity disorders in diabetics. J Res Health Sci. 2014;14(1):92-5.

Konin, Jeff, Denise Wiksten, Jerome Isear, and Holly Brader. Special tests for orthopedic examination. 3rd. Thoroare: SLACK Incorporated, 2006. Print.

Lee, Sang-Hun, MD, PhD, Eun-Seok Son, MD, PhD, Eun-Min Seo, MD, PhD, Kyung-Soo Suk, MD, PhD, Ki-Tack Kim, MD, PhD., Factors determining cervical spine sagittal balance in asymptomatic adults: correlation with spinopelvic balance and thoracic inlet alignment. The Spine Journal - (2013).

Link, Carol S, Garvice G Nicholson, Shirley A Shaddeau, Robert Birch and Marilyn R Gossman, Nicholson, Shirley A Shaddeau, Lumbar Curvature in Standing and Sitting in Two Types of Chairs: Relationship of Hamstring and Hip Flexor Muscle Length. *PHYS THER*. 1990; 70:611-618.

Lis, Angela Maria, Katia M. Black, Hayley Korn, Margareta Nordin, Association between sitting and occupational LBP. Eur Spine J (2007) 16:283–298.

Liu, Jing Z., Robert W. Brown, and Guang H. Yue, A Dynamical Model of Muscle Activation, Fatigue, and Recovery. Biophysical Journal Volume 82 May 2002 2344–2359.

Madeal, A.C. The Seated Man Homo Sedens. 2nd. Denmark: Dafnia Publications, 1983. Print.

Maiers, Michele, DC, MPH, Gert Bronfort, DC, PhD, Roni Evans, DC, MS, Jan Hartvigsen, DC, PhD, Kenneth Svendsen, MS, Yiscah Bracha, MS, Craig Schulz, DC, MS, Karen Schulz, DC, Richard Grimm, MD, PhD. Spinal manipulative therapy and exercise for seniors with chronic neck pain. The Spine Journal - (2014).

Makshsous, Mohsen, Fang Lin, James Bankard, Ronald W Hendrix, Matthew Hepler, Joel Press, Biomechanical effects of sitting with adjustable ischial and lumbar support on occupational low back pain: evaluation of sitting load and back muscle activity. *BMC Musculoskeletal Disorders* 2009, 10:17.

McArdle, William, Frank Katch, and Victor Katch. Exercise Physiology, Energy, Nutrition, and Human Performance. 3rd. Philadelphia: Lea & Febiger, 1991. Print.

McGill, S. (2007) LOW BACK Disorders Evidence Based Prevention and Rehabilitation 2nd edition. Champaign, IL. Human Kinetics.

McGill, Stuart M., PhD, Distribution of tissue loads the low back during a variety of daily and rehabilitation tasks. Journal of Rehabilitation Research and Development Vol. 34 No. 4, (1997) Pages 448-458.

McKenzie, Robin. *TREAT YOUR OWN BACK.* 6th. Waikanae: Spinal Productions, 1993. Print.

McKenzie, Robin. TREAT YOUR OWN NECK. 2nd. Waikanae: Spinal Productions, 1993. Print.

McMinn, R.M.H., Hutchings, R.T., Pegington, J. Abrahams, P. (1993) Mosby Year Book Inc. St. Louis, MO.

Nairn, Brian C., Stewart R. Chisholm, Janessa D.M. Drake, What is slumped sitting? A kinematic and electromyographical evaluation. Manual Therapy 18 (2013) 498-505.

Netter. Frank, H. (1992) Atlas of Human Anatomy. CIBA-GEIGY Corporation.

Norkin, Cynthia, and Pamela Levangie. JOINT STRUCTURE & FUNCTION. 10th. Philadelphia: F.A. Davis Company, 1990. Print.

O'Sullivan, Kieran, Peter O'Sullivan, Leonard O'Sullivan, Wim Dankaerts, What do physiotherapists consider to be the best sitting spinal posture? Manual Therapy 17 (2012) 432-437.

Owens, S. Christopher, Dale A. Gerke and Jean-Michel Brismée (2012). Ergonomic Impact of Spinal Loading and Recovery Positions on Intervertebral Disc Health: Strategies for Prevention and Management of Low Back Pain, Ergonomics - A Systems Approach, Dr. Isabel L. Nunes (Ed.), ISBN: 978-953-51-0601-2.

Prentice, William. Principles of Athletic Training, A Competency - Based Approach. Fifteenth. New York: McGraw-Hill, 2014. Print.

Quek June, Yong-Hao Pua, Ross A. Clark, Adam L. Bryant, Effects of thoracic kyphosis and forward head posture on cervical range of motion in older adults. Manual Therapy xxx (2012) 1-7.

Rohlmann, Antonius PhD, Thomas Zander, PhD, Friedmar Graichen, PhD, Marcel Dreischarf, MSc, Georg Bergmann, PhD. Measured loads on a vertebral body replacement during sitting. The Spine Journal 11 (2011) 870–87.5

Schinkel-Ivy, Alison, Brian C. Nairn, Janessa D.M. Drake, Investigation of trunk muscle co-contraction and its association with low back pain development during prolonged sitting. Journal of Electromyography and Kinesiology 23 (2013) 778–786.

Selvaraj, Israel. HUMAN POSTURE Good Health the Natural Way. 1st. Vanchioor: I. Selvaraj, 2005. Print.

Shi, Qiyun, Joy C MacDermid, Is surgical intervention more effective than non-surgical treatment for carpal tunnel syndrome? a systematic review. *Journal of Orthopaedic Surgery and Research* 2011, **6**:17.

Strong, Larkin L.; Zimmerman, Frederick J. Occupational Injury and Absence from Work Among African American, Hispanic, and Non-Hispanic White Workers in the National Longitudinal Survey of Youth. American Journal of Public Health. Jul2005, Vol. 95 Issue 7, p1226-1232. 7p. 3 Charts.

Thomsen, Jane F., Fred Gerr, Isam Atroshi, Carpal tunnel syndrome and the use of computer mouse and keyboard: A systematic review. **BMC Musculoskelet Disord. 2008; 9: 134.**

Tilley, Alvin, and Henry Dreyfuss. The MEASURE OF MAN AND WOMAN, HUMAN FACTORS IN DESIGN REVISED EDITION. New York: John Wiley & Sons, Inc., 2002. Print.

Tyson A.C. Beach, Robert J. Parkinson, J. Peter Stothart, PhD, Jack P. Callaghan, PhD., Effects of prolonged sitting on the passive flexion stiffness of the in vivo lumbar spine. The Spine Journal 5 (2005) 145–154.

Wang, Henry, Kaitlyn J. Weiss, Mason C. Haggerty, Jacqueline E. Heath, The effect of active sitting on trunk motion. Journal of Sport and Health Science xx (2014) 1-5.

Wilke, Hans–Joachim, PhD, Peter Neef, MD, Marco Caimi, MD, Thomas Hoogland, MD, and Lutz E. Claes, PhD., New *In Vivo* Measurements of Pressures in the Intervertebral Disc in Daily Life. SPINE Volume 24, Number 8, pp 755–762.

Wittink, H., R. Engelbert , T. Takken, The dangers of inactivity; exercise and inactivity physiology for the manual therapist. Manual Therapy 16 (2011) 209-216.

Xia, Ting, Laura A. Frey Law, A theoretical approach for modeling peripheral muscle fatigue and recovery. Journal of Biomechanics 41 (2008) 3046–3052.

<u>Online Resources:</u>

https://www.asam.org/docs/default-source/advocacy/opioid-addiction-disease-facts-figures.pdf

http://www.bls.gov/news.release/osh2.nr0.htm.

https://www.bls.gov/ooh/personal-care-and-service/fitness-trainers-and-instructors.htm

https://www.drugabuse.gov/about-nida/legislative-activities/testimony-to-congress/2016/americas-addiction-to-opioids-heroin-prescription-drug-abuse

https://en.wikipedia.org/wiki/Functional_training

https://en.wikipedia.org/wiki/High-intensity_interval_training

http://www.medicaldaily.com/stress-severe-pain-11-americans-suffer-chronic-pain-nih-states-347292

https://report.nih.gov/nihfactsheets/ViewFactSheet.aspx?csid=57

https://www.statista.com/statistics/236120/us-fitness-center-revenue/

https://www.statista.com/statistics/236123/us-fitness-center--health-club-memberships/

https://www.statista.com/topics/1141/health-and-fitness-clubs/